THE EVERYTHING ADDISON'S DISEASE DIET COOKBOOK

Nourishing Recipes for Thriving with Addison's disease Including Treatment, Prevention Strategies and Diet Plan

Joe Miller, RD

Copyright Page

Copyright © 2024 Joe Miller, RD

All rights reserved. No part of this publication may be reproduced, distributed, or transmitted in any form or by any means, including photocopying, recording, or other electronic or mechanical methods, without the prior written permission of the publisher, except in the case of brief quotation embodied in critical reviews and certain other non-commercial uses permitted by copyright law.

Table of Contents

Copyright Page 2

Table of Contents 3

INTRODUCTION 1

Comprehending Addison's Disease 4

What are the underlying factors that lead to Addison's Disease? 11

    Indications and Manifestations of Addison's Condition 16

    Diagnosing Addison's Disease 18

Strategies for Handling Addison's Disease 24

What It's Essential to Understand 30

    Actions to Take If You Are Afflicted with Addison's Disorder: 34

"Actions to Steer Clear of While Handling Addison's Condition:" 39

Recovery from Addison's disease 41

ADDISON DISEASE FRIENDLY DIET RECIPE IDEAS 44

ADDISON DISEASE FRIENDLY SODIUM-RICH RECIPES 44

Cauliflower Walnut Burritos 44

One Skillet Ground Beef Stroganoff 47

Garlic Broccoli Shrimp Stir Fry 50

Mushroom And Kale Burritos 52

Hearty Chicken Tortilla Soup 55

Baked Teriyaki Wings 59

Tofu Stir Fry 61

Sesame Peanut Noodles 64

Chipotle Chickpea Tacos 66

Creamy Broccoli Soup 67

Tofu Tacos 69

Ginger Mushroom Shrimp Stir-fry 71

Enchiladas Verdes Con Pollo As Made By Cuco 73

Tempeh Taco Salad 78

Sweet Potato Chicken Stir-fry With Peanut Sauce 81

Easy Chicken Cacciatore 85

Double Crunch Shrimp 88

Sweet Potato "Fried" Rice 92

Braised Chicken Thighs With Red Rice 94

Tofu Scramble Breakfast Tacos 98

Vegetarian Baked Beans 100

One-Pan Cider-Braised Pork Chops 103

Bánh Mì Bowl With Crispy Tofu 108

Tempeh Tacos 111

Stuffed Firecracker Chicken Rolls 113

Teriyaki Chicken Cauliflower Rice Bowl 116

Summertime Lentil Bolognese 119

Vegan Instant Pot Quinoa Chili 123

Korean-Style Bbq Beef Dinner Kit 126

Jazzy Shrimp And Grits 127

Chicken Tikka Masala Dinner Kit 131

Herb Sea Salt-Rubbed Chicken Thighs 133

Fajita Pasta Bake 135

Easily The Best Garlic Herb Roasted Potatoes 138

Spinach Artichoke Penne Pasta 141

Garlic Chicken Primavera 143

Chicken Fajita Quesadilla 145

Chinese Chicken Curry 148

Sun-Dried Tomato & Spinach Tuna Pasta 150

Chicken Teriyaki Chow Mein 151

ADDISON DISEASE FRIENDLY SOUP AND STEW RECIPES 156

Buffalo Cauliflower Nachos 156

Family Borscht Recipe By Andrew 159

Chicken And Kale Stew 162

Immunity Boosting Green Soup 167

Eggplant Potato Tomato Stew 171

Hearty Buffalo Chicken Soup 174

Hearty White Bean Stew 176

ADDISON DISEASE FRIENDLY SALAD RECIPES 180

Mushroom And Garlic Quinoa Salad 180

Tortilla Bowl Southwestern Salad 182

Roasted Veggie Quinoa Salad 185

Tuna Salad With Roasted Veggies 187

Roasted Cauliflower Salad 190

Sweet Potato And Chickpea Salad 193

Three Bean Salad 196

Chicken, Cranberry, And Pear Spinach Salad 198

Charred Summer Vegetable Salad 201

Farro Lentil Salad 204

Grilled Corn Summer Pasta Salad 207

Strawberry Poppy Seed Salad With Grilled Chicken 210

Avocado & Yogurt Chicken Salad 212

Hearty Roasted Veggie Salad 214

Roasted Sweet Potato And Apple Salad 217

Southwestern Salad 220

Buttermilk-fried Chicken Salad 222

Summer Vegetable Pesto Ribbon Salad 225

Ratatouille Salad 228

Kale & Sweet Potato Salad 231

Protein-Packed Roasted Vegetable Salad 234

Honey Mustard Chicken Salad 237

Avocado Quinoa Power Salad 240

In Summary 243

INTRODUCTION

Addison's disease, also known as adrenal insufficiency, is a relatively rare endocrine disorder that impacts approximately one in every 100,000 individuals. This condition does not discriminate based on gender or age, affecting both men and women equally across all age groups. Its symptoms include weight loss, muscular weakness, fatigue, low blood pressure, and occasionally, hyperpigmentation of the skin in exposed and unexposed areas of the body.

The hallmark of Addison's disease is the severe or complete deficiency of hormones produced in the adrenal cortex. Situated atop the kidneys, the adrenal glands play a crucial role in hormone production, particularly cortisol and aldosterone. When these hormones are insufficiently produced, the body loses salt and water through urine, leading to a dangerous drop in blood pressure. Additionally, potassium levels may rise to harmful levels, posing further health risks.

Despite ongoing research, effective treatment for Addison's disease remains elusive. Its impact on individuals extends beyond physical symptoms, as it may significantly restrict major life activities. According to the Americans with Disabilities Act (ADA), a person is considered disabled if they have a physical or mental impairment that substantially limits one or more major life activities, have a record of such an impairment, or are perceived to have such an impairment.

The ADA's definition underscores the profound impact Addison's disease can have on an individual's life, as it affects not only physical health but also social and occupational functioning. Given the complexity and variability of symptoms associated with Addison's disease, comprehensive support and accommodation are essential to ensuring affected individuals can navigate daily life with dignity and inclusion.

CHAPTER 1
Comprehending Addison's Disease

Addison's disease, an infrequent but significant endocrine malady, affects approximately one in every 100,000 individuals, presenting a unique confluence of factors that can precipitate its onset. This condition, known for its indiscriminate impact across genders and age groups, arises from a complex interplay of autoimmune dysregulation, infectious assaults, genetic predispositions, and iatrogenic insults inflicted upon the delicate adrenal glands.

The clinical presentation of Addison's disease encompasses a spectrum of symptoms, ranging from subtle to overt, and manifests as a constellation of physical and physiological disturbances. These include not only the hallmark manifestations of weight loss, muscular weakness, chronic fatigue, and hypotension but also the less conspicuous yet telling signs of skin hyperpigmentation observed in both sun-exposed and unexposed regions of the body. Such symptomatic diversity underscores the multifaceted nature of this disorder, rendering its diagnosis and management a nuanced endeavor.

At its core, Addison's disease derives its pathophysiological essence from the profound deficiency of cortisol and, in certain circumstances, aldosterone, key hormones meticulously crafted by the adrenal glands. This chronic insufficiency, also dubbed as hypocortisolism, plunges the body into a state of hormonal imbalance, eliciting cascades of physiological repercussions that reverberate throughout various organ systems.

Situated as sentinels atop the kidneys, the adrenal glands play a pivotal role in orchestrating the body's response to stress and maintaining metabolic equilibrium. The principal glucocorticoid, cortisol, wields a far-reaching influence, regulating diverse physiological processes ranging from immune modulation and inflammation suppression to glucose metabolism and protein synthesis. This hormone's indispensability to bodily homeostasis underscores the criticality of its precise regulation, a task entrusted to the intricate feedback loops orchestrated by the hypothalamus-pituitary-adrenal axis.

The intricate interplay between the hypothalamus, pituitary gland, and adrenal glands forms the backbone of cortisol regulation. The hypothalamus, perched atop the neuroendocrine hierarchy, initiates this regulatory dance by secreting releasing hormones that stimulate the pituitary gland to release adrenocorticotrophic hormone (ACTH). In response to ACTH, the adrenal glands dutifully churn out cortisol, which in turn signals the pituitary gland to curb ACTH secretion, thus completing the feedback loop.

Yet, Addison's disease doesn't confine its disruption solely to cortisol production; it also encroaches upon aldosterone synthesis, further complicating the body's delicate electrolyte balance and blood pressure regulation. Aldosterone, a mineralocorticoid hormone, exerts its influence by orchestrating sodium and potassium reabsorption in the kidneys, thereby modulating blood volume and pressure. Inadequate aldosterone production heralds a cascade of fluid and electrolyte imbalances, accentuating the clinical complexity of Addison's disease.

In the labyrinthine landscape of endocrine disorders, Addison's disease emerges as a poignant reminder of the intricate interplay between genetic predispositions, environmental triggers, and immunological derangements. Its clinical heterogeneity underscores the imperative for a comprehensive understanding of its etiopathogenesis, heralding a new era of personalized diagnostics and therapeutics aimed at mitigating its multifaceted impact on affected individuals.

CHAPTER 2

What are the underlying factors that lead to Addison's Disease?

The condition of adrenal insufficiency, characterized by the inadequate production of cortisol, can stem from a diverse array of underlying causes, each contributing to the intricate tapestry of hormonal dysregulation. This deficiency may originate from abnormalities within the adrenal glands themselves, referred to as primary adrenal insufficiency, or from deficiencies in the production of adrenocorticotropic hormone (ACTH) by the pituitary gland, termed secondary adrenal insufficiency.

Primary adrenal insufficiency predominantly arises from autoimmune processes, where the body's immune system mounts an assault on the adrenal cortex, leading to its gradual destruction. This autoimmune phenomenon accounts for approximately 70% of documented cases of Addison's disease, a subset of adrenal insufficiency wherein the adrenal cortex's destruction exceeds 90%. Consequently, deficiencies in both glucocorticoid and mineralocorticoid hormones become prevalent, disrupting essential physiological functions.

The spectrum of primary adrenal insufficiency encompasses various clinical entities, including Type I and Type II polyendocrine insufficiency syndromes, each characterized by distinct clinical features and associated comorbidities. While Type

I polyendocrine insufficiency syndrome manifests predominantly in younger individuals, Type II, also known as Schmidt's syndrome, tends to affect a broader demographic, often presenting with a constellation of endocrine abnormalities.

In affluent nations, tuberculosis (TB) historically served as a significant etiological factor, contributing to nearly a fifth of primary adrenal insufficiency cases. However, advancements in TB therapy have significantly reduced the incidence of adrenal insufficiency related to TB infections of the adrenal glands. Nonetheless, chronic infections, fungal invasions, metastatic malignancies, amyloidosis, and surgical interventions on the adrenal glands remain less common yet noteworthy triggers of primary adrenal insufficiency, underscoring the multifactorial nature of this condition.

Secondary adrenal insufficiency, on the other hand, arises from deficiencies in ACTH production by the pituitary gland, leading to decreased cortisol synthesis while sparing aldosterone production. This form of adrenal insufficiency often arises secondary to prolonged administration of exogenous glucocorticoid hormones, such as prednisone, which suppress the hypothalamic-pituitary-adrenal axis. Inflammatory conditions like rheumatoid arthritis, asthma, and ulcerative colitis, for which glucocorticoids are commonly prescribed, further exacerbate this phenomenon by inhibiting the production of corticotropin-releasing hormone (CRH) and subsequently ACTH.

Additionally, surgical removal of benign ACTH-producing pituitary tumors or disruptions in the hypothalamic-pituitary axis due to tumors, infections, vascular insufficiency, radiation therapy, or surgical interventions can precipitate secondary adrenal insufficiency. The cessation of ACTH secretion or compromised blood supply to the pituitary gland can disrupt the delicate hormonal balance, necessitating prompt recognition and intervention to restore physiological equilibrium. Thus, the intricate interplay of endocrine dysregulation and environmental triggers underscores the complexity of adrenal insufficiency, prompting a nuanced approach to its diagnosis and management.

Indications and Manifestations of Addison's Condition

Due to the prevalence of symptoms such as fatigue, lack of energy, weight loss, and nausea, Addison's disease often progresses slowly and can be challenging to pinpoint. A notable distinguishing feature in some individuals with pituitary conditions that cause excessive ACTH release is the occurrence of skin darkening (pigmentation) in specific areas. This darkening tends to manifest on sun-exposed regions like the hands, as well as on the lining of the lips, the creases on the palms, and any recent scars.

The most common symptoms include weakness, fatigue, loss of appetite, nausea, weight reduction, skin discoloration, and low blood pressure, particularly upon standing (known as postural or orthostatic hypotension), resulting in dizziness and fainting.

The Addisonian Crisis represents a dire scenario characterized by severe and abrupt symptom onset. Patients experience plummeting blood pressure (hypotension), accompanied by nausea, vomiting, abdominal discomfort, and often an inexplicable fever. This constitutes a hazardous situation, necessitating prompt administration of cortisol therapy following blood sample collection. The Addisonian crisis can arise due to various triggers, such as hemorrhage within the adrenal glands or stressful events like trauma, surgery, or infection. Recognizing the signs and swiftly initiating appropriate intervention is paramount in managing this life-threatening complication.

Diagnosing Addison's Disease

The early detection of adrenal insufficiency poses a formidable challenge, often requiring a comprehensive evaluation of a patient's medical history to unveil subtle clues, such as the telltale darkening of the skin, which can arouse suspicion of Addison's disease. Diagnostic endeavors in this realm typically pivot around biochemical laboratory investigations aimed at unraveling the enigmatic nature of this condition. The overarching goal of such tests is twofold: firstly, to discern the presence of inadequate cortisol levels and subsequently to decipher the underlying etiology driving this deficiency. Complementary to these efforts, imaging modalities like X-rays offer valuable insights into the structural integrity of the adrenal and pituitary glands, furnishing clinicians with vital clues in their diagnostic odyssey.

Among the pantheon of diagnostic tools, the ACTH Stimulation Examination reigns supreme as the gold standard for unmasking Addison's disease. This meticulously orchestrated test involves the administration of a synthetic derivative of ACTH, followed by the measurement of cortisol levels in the blood and/or urine before and after the hormonal stimulus. The body's natural response to ACTH injection typically entails a surge in cortisol levels; however, patients afflicted with adrenal insufficiency may exhibit either a blunted or absent response. In cases where the results of the short ACTH stimulation test prove inconclusive, a protracted evaluation spanning 48 to 72 hours becomes imperative to delineate the underlying cause of adrenal insufficiency.

Furthermore, in scenarios where the specter of an Addisonian crisis looms large, prompt therapeutic intervention assumes paramount importance, necessitating the administration of saline, fluids, and glucocorticoid hormones to stave off impending catastrophe. While the definitive diagnosis remains elusive amidst the tumult of acute management, serial monitoring of blood ACTH and cortisol levels during the crisis and post-therapy suffices to delineate the underlying pathology. Once the crisis abates and pharmacotherapy ceases, a temporary hiatus in further diagnostic pursuits ensues, allowing for a more accurate assessment to ensue after the dust settles.

In addition to the ACTH Stimulation Examination, the insulin-induced hypoglycemia test emerges as a stalwart diagnostic ally, offering invaluable insights into the interplay between the hypothalamus, pituitary, and adrenal glands in response to stress. This dynamic test involves sequential blood sampling to gauge glucose and cortisol levels before and after the administration of rapidly acting insulin, shedding light on the body's capacity to mount a robust hormonal response in the face of physiological perturbation.

Moreover, ancillary diagnostic endeavors like abdominal X-rays serve as indispensable adjuncts in the diagnostic armamentarium, enabling clinicians to discern the presence of calcium deposits within the adrenal glands, a harbinger of conditions like tuberculosis. Similarly, advanced imaging modalities such as CT scans afford a nuanced appraisal of the pituitary gland's structure and function, offering invaluable insights into the etiological underpinnings of secondary adrenal insufficiency.

In the intricate tapestry of diagnostic endeavors, Addison's disease emerges as a complex clinical entity, necessitating a multifaceted approach to unravel its cryptic manifestations. By leveraging a diverse array of diagnostic tools and techniques, clinicians can navigate the labyrinthine terrain of adrenal insufficiency with confidence, ensuring timely intervention and optimized patient outcomes.

CHAPTER 3
Strategies for Handling Addison's Disease

The treatment protocol for Addison's disease revolves around compensating for the deficient hormones that the adrenal glands fail to produce. This comprehensive approach involves the administration of synthetic replacements to restore hormonal balance and mitigate the myriad symptoms associated with this condition.

Hydrocortisone pills, a synthetic glucocorticoid, serve as the cornerstone of therapy, taken orally once or twice daily to replenish cortisol levels. In cases where aldosterone deficiency is also present, daily oral doses of fludrocortisone acetate

(Florinef), a mineralocorticoid, are prescribed to address the electrolyte imbalance. Additionally, patients undergoing aldosterone replacement therapy are typically advised to increase their salt intake to offset the potential sodium loss associated with the condition.

For individuals with secondary adrenal insufficiency, wherein aldosterone production remains intact, aldosterone replacement therapy is not required, underscoring the tailored nature of treatment plans tailored to each patient's unique needs.

In situations necessitating immediate intervention, such as addisonian crises characterized by dangerously low blood pressure, hypoglycemia, or hyperkalemia, intravenous injections of hydrocortisone, saline, and dextrose are administered promptly to restore physiological equilibrium. This emergent therapy typically yields rapid and pronounced results, facilitating the transition to maintenance therapy once the patient can resume oral medication intake.

However, certain unique scenarios, such as surgical interventions or pregnancy, demand specialized considerations in the management of Addison's disease. Patients undergoing surgery necessitating general anesthesia receive preemptive injections of hydrocortisone and saline the night before the procedure, continuing until they regain consciousness and can resume oral medications. Similarly, pregnant women with primary adrenal insufficiency receive conventional replacement therapy, with adjustments made as necessary to accommodate the physiological changes associated with pregnancy.

Education and preparedness play pivotal roles in empowering patients to manage Addison's disease effectively. Patients are instructed on the importance of carrying identification specifying their medical condition, along with instructions for emergency responders on administering cortisol in the event of incapacitation. Moreover, they are advised to maintain a readily accessible emergency kit containing needles, syringes, and injectable cortisol for use during stressful situations or illnesses that may precipitate adrenal crises.

Furthermore, meticulous attention is paid to preventive measures, such as wearing medical alert bracelets or necklaces to alert emergency services of the patient's medical condition, particularly during instances where the patient may be unable to communicate their medical history. These proactive measures serve as invaluable safeguards, ensuring timely access to appropriate medical care in critical situations.

CHAPTER 4
What It's Essential to Understand

The historical narrative of Addison's disease finds its genesis in the meticulous observations of Thomas Addison, who first documented the condition in 1855. In its nascent stages, tuberculosis (TB) stood as the predominant catalyst behind adrenal gland destruction, ushering in an era where the malady was synonymous with TB-induced adrenal insufficiency. However, the landscape of modern endocrinology has witnessed a paradigm shift, with autoimmune aggression emerging as the primary etiological culprit in the majority of Addison's disease cases, relegating tuberculosis to a relatively uncommon cause. Other adrenal disorders and infiltrations, while existent, remain uncommon triggers for the onset of this ailment.

Epidemiological assessments paint a picture of Addison's disease prevalence hovering between 40 to 60 cases per million individuals, with an annual incidence of 3 to 4 new cases per million. This relatively low prevalence underscores the rarity of this endocrine disorder within the broader medical landscape.

The pathophysiological underpinnings of Addison's disease are rooted in the deficiency of both cortisol and aldosterone, distinct from adrenocorticotropic hormone (ACTH) deficiency, where the mineralocorticoid axis typically remains intact. Consequently, clinical manifestations often manifest as a trifecta of weariness, malaise, and skin pigmentation alterations induced by elevated

ACTH levels, culminating eventually in the ominous specter of adrenal or Addisonian crisis.

The clinical milieu of Addison's disease crisis is typified by biochemical perturbations, with hyponatremia, hyperkalemia, and dehydration emerging as recurrent biochemical hallmarks. However, it's noteworthy that these biochemical aberrations may not always manifest in symptomatic individuals who are not experiencing a crisis.

Diagnosis of Addison's disease necessitates a judicious amalgamation of clinical acumen and investigative prowess, often relying on basal cortisol levels, synacthen tests, and ancillary investigations to discern primary from secondary adrenal insufficiency etiologies. Ancillary investigations such as ACTH, renin, adrenal antibodies, and tests assessing other pituitary functions play pivotal roles in elucidating the underlying pathophysiology.

Management of Addison's disease revolves around the judicious administration of glucocorticoid and mineralocorticoid replacement therapy, typically in the form of thrice-daily hydrocortisone and fludrocortisone, respectively. Equally paramount is patient education regarding self-adjustment of steroid replacement dosages during acute intercurrent illnesses, ensuring optimal management and mitigation of adrenal crisis risks.

The advent of modified release formulations of hydrocortisone holds promise in refining therapeutic outcomes, although regulatory clearance hurdles persist, casting a veil of uncertainty over their clinical utility. Vigilant monitoring and therapeutic titration remain the cornerstones of effective Addison's disease management, emblematic of the intricate dance between medical science and clinical pragmatism in navigating the labyrinthine landscape of endocrine disorders.

Actions to Take If You Are Afflicted with Addison's Disorder:

- Regular Consultations with your Healthcare Provider: It is highly advisable to schedule frequent appointments with your doctor to ensure proper monitoring and management of your condition. These regular check-ins allow your healthcare team to assess your progress, adjust your treatment plan if necessary, and address any concerns or questions you may have.

• Adherence to Medication Regimen: Strict adherence to your prescribed medication regimen is paramount for effectively managing Addison's disease. Always take your medications exactly as directed by your doctor, and do not alter your dosage or frequency without consulting them first.

• Precautions Prior to Surgical Procedures or Medication Changes: Before undergoing any surgical procedures or starting new prescription medications, it is imperative to discuss these plans with your healthcare provider. Changes in medication or surgical interventions may necessitate adjustments to your treatment plan to ensure optimal health outcomes.

- Medical Alert Bracelet: Carrying a medical alert bracelet or necklace is strongly recommended for individuals with Addison's disease. This can provide crucial information to medical professionals in the event of an emergency, alerting them to your condition and any specific medical needs or considerations.

- Emergency Medication Kit: It is prudent to keep an emergency medication kit readily accessible in case of adrenal crisis. Ensure that both you and your family members are familiar with how to administer these medications, and regularly check the expiration dates to ensure their efficacy.

• Stress Management: Efforts to minimize stress in your daily life are essential for managing Addison's disease effectively. Engage in relaxation techniques, mindfulness practices, or hobbies that promote mental and emotional well-being to help mitigate the impact of stress on your health.

• Healthy Lifestyle Choices: Maintaining a balanced lifestyle is key to supporting overall health and well-being. Consume alcohol in moderation, follow a well-rounded diet rich in essential nutrients, including an adequate intake of sodium, and incorporate regular physical activity into your routine, ensuring to strike a balance and avoid excessive exertion.

- Monitoring Symptoms and Seeking Medical Attention: Pay close attention to any changes in your health status and promptly report any concerning symptoms to your healthcare provider. Symptoms such as nausea, vomiting, fever, unexplained weight loss, weakness, or exhaustion may indicate a worsening of your condition and require immediate medical evaluation.

- Gradual Medication Adjustment: If approved by your doctor, any adjustments to your medication dosage should be made gradually and under their supervision. This approach helps minimize the risks associated with medication changes, such as weight gain, diabetes, or hypertension, ensuring a safe and effective management strategy for Addison's disease.

"Actions to Steer Clear of While Handling Addison's Condition:"

1. Refrain from excessive consumption of potassium-rich foods such as bananas, oranges, and salt substitutes to avoid potential complications stemming from potassium overdose. While these foods are nutritious in moderation, overindulgence can lead to imbalances in electrolytes, posing risks to cardiovascular and neuromuscular function. It's essential to maintain a balanced diet that includes a

variety of foods while being mindful of potassium intake levels.

2. Ensure strict adherence to medication schedules and avoid missing any prescribed doses. Consistency in medication adherence is paramount for managing conditions effectively, including Addison's disease. Skipping doses or irregular medication intake can disrupt hormone levels, exacerbate symptoms, and compromise overall health outcomes. Establishing a routine and utilizing reminder tools can help maintain medication compliance and optimize therapeutic efficacy. Remember, adherence to treatment plans is crucial for achieving and sustaining health improvements.

Recovery from Addison's disease

To ensure your safety and well-being while managing Addison's disease, it is imperative to take proactive measures and maintain open communication with healthcare professionals. One such precautionary step involves carrying a medical alert card or wearing a bracelet that clearly identifies your condition. These identifiers serve as vital indicators to emergency personnel, providing crucial information about your health status and required medical interventions in case of unforeseen emergencies.

Furthermore, it is prudent to always have additional medication readily accessible, particularly when embarking on travels or engaging in activities away from home. This precautionary measure mitigates the risk of medication shortages or unexpected delays in accessing necessary treatments. Additionally, it is advisable to keep a needle and injectable form of your medication on hand at all times. This ensures preparedness to administer emergency doses promptly, should the need arise.

Maintaining regular communication and follow-ups with your healthcare provider is paramount in effectively managing Addison's disease. Your doctor plays a pivotal role in overseeing your treatment regimen, monitoring your health status, and adjusting medication dosages as needed to optimize therapeutic outcomes. By staying in touch with your healthcare team, you can stay informed about the latest advancements in Addison's disease management and receive personalized guidance tailored to your specific needs and circumstances.

In summary, vigilance, preparedness, and proactive communication with healthcare professionals are essential components of effectively managing Addison's disease. By adhering to these guidelines and taking proactive measures to safeguard your health, you can navigate the challenges posed by this condition with confidence and resilience.

CHAPTER 5
ADDISON DISEASE FRIENDLY DIET RECIPE IDEAS

ADDISON DISEASE FRIENDLY SODIUM-RICH RECIPES

Cauliflower Walnut Burritos

Ingredients Needed

for 4 servings

½ head cauliflower, broken into florets

¾ cup walnuts (75 g)

olive oil, to taste

½ medium yellow onion, diced

2 cloves garlic, minced

2 ½ teaspoons chili powder

1 teaspoon ground cumin

½ teaspoon smoked paprika

2 tablespoons low sodium soy sauce

¼ cup low sodium vegetable broth (60 mL)

kosher salt, to taste

pepper, to taste

4 large flour tortillas

2 cups spanish rice (460 g), cooked

lettuce, chopped, for serving

tomato, diced, for serving

shredded vegan cheddar cheese, for serving

guacamole, for serving

How To Prepare :

Add the cauliflower florets and walnuts to a food processor and pulse until crumbly. Set aside.

Heat a drizzle of olive oil in a large saucepan over medium heat. Once the oil begins to shimmer, add the onion and cook for 3-4 minutes, until semi-translucent. Add the cauliflower mixture and cook for 4-5 minutes, until the cauliflower is semi-tender.

Add another drizzle of olive oil, the garlic, chili powder, cumin, paprika, and soy sauce and cook for 2-3 minutes more, until the spices are fragrant. Add the vegetable broth and cook for another 5-6 minutes, until the broth has evaporated and the cauliflower is tender. Season with salt and pepper to taste.

To assemble a burrito, add ¼ of the Spanish rice, ¼ of the cauliflower-walnut mixture, some lettuce, tomatoes, vegan cheese, and guacamole to the center of a tortilla. Fold in the sides and roll up, keeping the filling tucked in place. Repeat with the remaining ingredients. Cut in half and serve.

Enjoy!

One Skillet Ground Beef Stroganoff

Ingredients Needed

for 4 servings

1 tablespoon olive oil

8 oz white button mushroom (225 g), sliced

2 tablespoons butter

½ onion, diced

1 lb ground beef (455 g)

2 teaspoons garlic powder

3 tablespoons flour

1 teaspoon paprika

¼ cup dry sherry (60 mL)

4 cups low sodium beef broth (945 mL)

1 ½ teaspoons salt

½ teaspoon pepper

4 cups dry egg noodle (400 g)

½ cup sour cream (115 g)

2 tablespoons fresh parsley, chopped

How To Prepare :

Add olive to a large pan over medium heat. Once the oil begins to shimmer, add the mushrooms and cook until tender, 5 to 6 minutes. Transfer the mushrooms to a plate.

In the same pan, add the butter. Add the onion, ground beef, and garlic powder. Stir until the meat is browned, breaking it up as you stir.

Drain any excess fat and return the pan to the stove.

Add the flour and paprika. Stir until thick, about 1 to 2 minutes.

Add the sherry, and stir, scraping up any brown bits from the bottom of the pan.

Add the beef broth and bring the mixture to a boil.

Add the egg noodles, salt, and pepper. Reduce the heat to simmer. Cover the pan with a lid.

Stir often, until the noodles are tender, about 8 to 10 minutes.

Return the mushrooms to the pan and stir to combine.

Add the sour cream and stir. Top with chopped parsley.

Enjoy!

Garlic Broccoli Shrimp Stir Fry

Ingredients Needed

for 4 servings

1 lb large shrimp (455 g), peeled and deveined

3 cloves garlic, minced

2 cups broccoli floret (500 g)

½ onion, diced

1 tablespoon low sodium soy sauce

2 tablespoons sesame oil, divided

½ teaspoon salt, divided

How To Prepare :

Heat 1 tablespoon of sesame oil in a large, nonstick skillet over medium heat.

Pour in the shrimp and season with ¼ teaspoon of the salt.

Fry the shrimp for 1 minute on each side.

Remove the shrimp from the pan and pour in the remaining 1 tablespoon of oil.

Toss in the onion and remaining ¼ teaspoon of salt and sauté for a few minutes until they begin to soften.

Add in the broccoli, garlic and soy sauce and sauté until the garlic is fragrant, about 30 seconds.

Toss the shrimp back into the pan and mix until everything is well incorporated and the shrimp is fully cooked, about 1 minute.

Divide the mixture evenly between 4 bowls.

Enjoy!

Mushroom And Kale Burritos

Ingredients

for 2 servings

olive oil, to taste

10 oz cremini mushroom (285 g), sliced

2 cloves garlic, minced, divided

½ teaspoon smoked paprika

2 tablespoons low sodium soy sauce, divided

¼ teaspoon liquid smoke

kosher salt, to taste

pepper, to taste

½ medium yellow onion, sliced

5 cups curly kale (500 g), chopped

¼ cup low sodium vegetable broth (60 mL)

red pepper flake, to taste

1 cup brown rice (230 g), cooked

2 large flour tortillas

How To Prepare :

Heat a drizzle of olive oil in a large saucepan. Once the oil begins to shimmer, add the mushrooms and cook for 4-5 minutes, until most of their liquid has been released. Add a bit more olive oil, 1 clove of garlic, the paprika, 1 tablespoon soy sauce, and the liquid smoke and cook for 3-4 more minutes, until the mushrooms are golden brown. Season with salt and pepper to taste. Remove from pan and set aside.

To the same pan, add another drizzle of olive oil and the onion. Cook for 3-4 minutes, until the onion is semi-translucent. Add the kale and vegetable broth. Cover and steam for 5 minutes, or until the kale has wilted by about 75 percent.

Add another drizzle of olive oil, the remaining clove of garlic, red pepper flakes, remaining tablespoon of soy sauce, and pepper and cook for 2-3 minutes, until the garlic is fragrant.

To assemble a burrito, add ½ of the brown rice, ½ of the kale mixture, and ½ of the mushrooms to the center of a tortilla. Fold in the sides and roll up, keeping the filling tucked in place. Repeat with the remaining ingredients. Cut in half and serve.

Enjoy!

Hearty Chicken Tortilla Soup

Ingredients

for 8 servings

8 oz large white onion (225 g), roughly chopped

6 cloves garlic

1 jalapeño, seeded and roughly chopped

1 chipotle pepper in adobo sauce, to taste

1 cup fresh cilantro (40 g), loosely packed

4 roma tomatoes, roughly chopped

1 lb boneless, skinless chicken thighs (455 g)

kosher salt, to taste

1 teaspoon dried oregano

2 tablespoons olive oil, divided

8 cups low sodium chicken stock (2 L)

25 oz hominy (625 g), drained and rinsed

2 red bell peppers, seeded and chopped

¼ cup lime juice (60 mL)

For Serving

onion, finely chopped

fresh cilantro

avocado, thinly sliced

cotija cheese, crumbled

tortilla strip

lime wedge

How To Prepare :

Add the onion, garlic, jalapeño, chipotle peppers, cilantro, and tomatoes to a food processor. Puree until well combined, with no large pieces remaining, about 2 minutes. Set aside.

Season the chicken thighs on both sides with salt and the oregano.

In a large pot, heat 1 tablespoon of olive oil over medium-high heat. Sear the chicken thighs for 4-5 minutes on each side, until golden brown. Transfer to a cutting board. Shred the chicken using 2 forks. Set aside.

Add the remaining tablespoon of olive oil to the same pot if it appears dry. Pour the reserved puree into the pot. Cook over medium-high heat for 10 minutes, until the liquid has started to evaporate.

Reduce the heat to medium and continue cooking until nearly all the moisture has been cooked out and the puree has reduced to a dark paste, stirring occasionally to prevent burning, about 20 minutes.

Pour in the chicken stock and stir, scraping the bottom of the pan to incorporate any browned bits. Increase the heat to medium-high. Stir in the shredded chicken and bring to a simmer.

Once the stock is simmering, stir in the hominy and bell pepper. Reduce the heat to medium and simmer for 5-10 minutes to allow the flavors to meld. Add the lime juice and season with salt to taste.

Serve the soup hot, with onion, cilantro, avocado, cotija cheese, tortilla strips, and lime wedges alongside for topping.

Enjoy!

Baked Teriyaki Wings

Ingredients

for 2 servings

1 lb chicken wings (455 g)

2 teaspoons baking powder

1 teaspoon salt

Teriyaki Sauce

⅓ cup low sodium soy sauce (70 mL)

2 tablespoons honey

2 tablespoons brown sugar

1 tablespoon sesame seed

How To Prepare :

Preheat oven to 400°F/200°C.

Remove excess moisture from chicken wings with a paper towel.

In a large bowl, stir in baking powder and salt until chicken is thoroughly coated.

Bake on a baking rack for 1 hour, or until golden brown and crispy, flipping every 20 minutes. (For best results, place baking rack on a baking sheet covered with parchment paper or foil to catch drippings).

In a skillet, combine soy sauce, honey, and brown sugar on medium heat. Bring to a boil and add in sesame seeds.

Once sauce is thickened, stir in chicken wings until fully coated.

Serve with your favorite side dish or dipping sauce.

Enjoy!

Tofu Stir Fry

Ingredients Needed

for 2 servings

4 cloves garlic, minced, divided

2 teaspoons fresh ginger, grated

1 tablespoon honey

1 teaspoon sriracha

¼ cup lime juice (60 mL)

¼ cup reduced sodium soy sauce (60 mL)

1 block extra firm tofu

2 tablespoons sesame oil

1 cup sliced white onion

1 cup sliced carrot

1 cup sliced red bell pepper

½ cup edamame (75 g), frozen, thawed

3 cups soba noodle (300 g), cooked

1 tablespoon sesame seed

green onion, chopped, to serve

How To Prepare :

In a medium bowl, mix together 2 cloves of garlic, the ginger, honey, Sriracha, lime juice, and soy sauce. Set aside.

Wrap the tofu in a dish towel, then place a plate on top. Let drain for 10-15 minutes, then remove the plate, unwrap the tofu, and slice into cubes.

In a wok or large frying pan, heat the sesame oil over medium heat. Add the tofu and pan fry for 5-7 minutes, stirring occasionally.

Add the remaining 2 cloves of minced garlic and the onion and stir until softened, about 1 minute.

Add the carrot, bell pepper, and edamame and cook, stirring occasionally, until tender, 2-3 minutes.

Add the soba noodles, reserved sauce, and sesame seeds. Cook for 1-2 minutes, stirring occasionally, until warmed through. Remove the pan from the heat.

Garnish with green onions, if desired.

Enjoy!

Sesame Peanut Noodles

Ingredients

for 4 servings

½ cup peanut butter (120 g)

3 tablespoons low sodium soy sauce

2 tablespoons sesame oil

2 tablespoons rice vinegar

3 tablespoons water

2 ½ teaspoons brown sugar

1 clove garlic

½ tablespoon fresh ginger, minced

8 oz spaghetti (240 g), cooked according to package instructions

½ cup shredded carrot (55 g)

½ cup shredded red cabbage (50 g)

¾ cup edamame (115 g), shelled

peanut, for garnish

1 tablespoon black sesame seeds, for garnish

scallion, sliced, for garnish

How To Prepare :

In a blender, combine the peanut butter, soy sauce, sesame oil, rice vinegar, water, brown sugar, garlic, and ginger and blend until smooth.

In a large bowl, add the spaghetti, carrots, cabbage, and edamame and pour over the peanut sauce. Use tongs to mix well, until sauce is fully incorporated.

Transfer to bowls and top with peanuts, black sesame seeds, and scallion.

Enjoy!

Chipotle Chickpea Tacos

Ingredients

for 2 servings

1 tablespoon olive oil

15 oz chickpeas (425 g), 1 can, drained and rinsed

2 tablespoons low sodium soy sauce

1 teaspoon chipotle chili powder

1 teaspoon garlic powder

tortilla, to serve

How To Prepare :

Add the olive oil to a pan over medium heat. Once the oil begins to shimmer, add the chickpeas and cook until slightly golden, stirring occasionally.

Add soy sauce, chipotle chili powder, and garlic powder to the chickpeas and sauté for 3-4 more minutes, until golden brown.

Serve on warm tortillas with desired taco toppings.

Enjoy!

Creamy Broccoli Soup

Ingredients Needed

for 8 servings

1 tablespoon olive oil

1 small onion, diced

3 garlics, minced

1 teaspoon kosher salt

½ teaspoon pepper

2 cups mashed potato (500 g)

2 small heads broccoli, including stems, chopped

2 ½ cups low sodium vegetable broth (600 mL)

2 ½ cups milk (600 mL), of your choice

¼ teaspoon ground nutmeg

How To Prepare :

Heat the olive oil in a large pot over medium heat. Once the oil begins to shimmer, add the onion and cook for 3-4 minutes, until semi-translucent. Add the garlic, salt, and pepper and cook for 2-3 minutes more, until the garlic is fragrant.

Add the mashed potatoes, broccoli, vegetable broth, and milk and bring to a boil. Cover and reduce the heat to low. Simmer for 20 minutes, or until the broccoli is tender.

Use an immersion blender to blend the soup until smooth.

Stir in the nutmeg, then ladle into bowls.

Enjoy!

Tofu Tacos

Ingredients

for 2 servings

14 oz extra firm tofu (395 g), 1 block, drained

3 tablespoons low sodium soy sauce

¼ cup tomato sauce (65 g)

2 teaspoons chili powder

2 teaspoons garlic powder

1 teaspoon cumin

½ teaspoon black pepper

1 pinch cayenne

olive oil, for drizzling

4 small corn tortillas

Toppings

lettuce, shredded

tomato, diced

vegan shredded cheese, or regular

guacamole

How To Prepare :

Preheat the oven to 400°F (200°C).

Use your hands to crumble the tofu into a medium bowl. Add the soy sauce, tomato sauce, chili powder, garlic powder, cumin, pepper, and cayenne and stir until well-combined.

Add a drizzle of olive oil to a large baking sheet. Transfer the tofu to the baking sheet, using a spatula to spread it out as much as possible.

Bake for 20-25 minutes, stirring halfway through, until golden brown and slightly crispy.

Fill the tortillas with the tofu, lettuce, tomato, shredded cheese, and guacamole.

Enjoy!

Ginger Mushroom Shrimp Stir-fry

Ingredients Needed

for 4 servings

2 tablespoons sesame oil

1 lb large shrimp (455 g), peeled and deveined

½ teaspoon salt, divided

2 cups mushroom (150 g), sliced

1 cup asparagus (125 g), sliced

1 tablespoon ginger, minced

1 tablespoon low sodium soy sauce

How To Prepare :

Heat 1 tablespoon of sesame oil in a large, non-stick skillet over medium heat. Add the shrimp and season with ¼ teaspoon of salt. Cook the shrimp for 1 minute on each side, until just pink. Remove from the pan.

Add the remaining tablespoon of oil to the pan. Toss in the mushrooms, asparagus, and remaining

¼ teaspoon of salt and sauté for a few minutes, until the vegetables begin to soften.

Add the ginger and soy sauce and sauté until the ginger is fragrant, about 30 seconds.

Toss the shrimp back into the pan and mix until everything is well incorporated and the shrimp is fully cooked, about 1 minute.

Divide the mixture evenly between 4 bowls.

Enjoy!

Enchiladas Verdes Con Pollo As Made By Cuco

Ingredients

for 6 servings

1 lb medium tomatillo (455 g), husks removed

½ medium white onion, halved

1 serrano pepper, stemmed

3 cloves garlic

water, as needed

½ bunch fresh cilantro, leaves and soft stems roughly chopped, plus more leaves for garnish - about 1 cup (40 G)

1 tablespoon kosher salt

½ cup low sodium chicken stock (120 mL)

¼ cup vegetable oil (60 mL), divided

12 thick slices corn tortilla

3 cups shredded rotisserie chicken (375 g)

5 oz queso fresco (150 g), crumbled

¼ medium white onion, finely chopped, for garnish

2 tablespoons mexican crema, for garnish

How To Prepare :

Add the tomatillos, onion, serrano peppers, and garlic to a medium saucepan. Pour in enough water to just cover. Bring to a boil over medium-high heat and cook until the vegetables are very tender and the tomatillos have changed color, 8–10 minutes.

Use a slotted spoon to transfer the cooked vegetables to a blender and discard the cooking liquid. Purée the vegetables until broken down. Add the chopped cilantro, salt, and chicken stock. Blend the salsa until smooth. It should be speckled and thick.

Heat 2 tablespoons of vegetable oil in a large pan over medium-high heat. When the oil is shimmering, add the salsa verde to the pan. Bring to a boil, then reduce the heat to maintain a strong simmer. Cook until the salsa deepens in color and thickens slightly, about 10 minutes, stirring occasionally. Pour the salsa into a medium bowl and set aside. Wipe out the pan with a paper towel.

Heat the remaining 2 tablespoons of vegetable oil in the same pan over medium-high heat. Working 2 at a time, fry the tortillas for 1 minute per side, until starting to brown but not completely fried. They should be crisp around the edges but still pliable enough to roll. Transfer the tortillas to a paper towel-lined baking sheet to drain.

Set a rack in the center of the oven and turn on the broiler.

Spread ½ cup of the salsa verde over the bottom of a 9 x 13-inch (22 x 33 cm) baking dish.

Assemble the enchiladas: Dip a tortilla in the remaining salsa verde so both sides are coated. Place the tortilla on a flat surface and add about 4 tablespoons of shredded chicken to the center. Roll tightly. Place the filled tortilla, seam-side down, in the baking dish. Repeat with the remaining ingredients.

Pour any remaining salsa over the top of the enchiladas, then sprinkle with the queso fresco.

Broil the enchiladas until the cheese is just melted, 2–4 minutes.

Serve the enchiladas warm with the diced onion, Mexican crema, and cilantro leaves for topping

Enjoy!

Tempeh Taco Salad

Ingredients Needed

for 3 servings

Tempeh

8 oz tempeh (225 g), 1 package

olive oil, for cooking

3 tablespoons low sodium soy sauce

2 teaspoons garlic powder

2 teaspoons chili powder

1 teaspoon cumin

Avocado Dressing

1 avocado

1 lime, juiced

¼ cup olive oil (60 mL)

salt, to taste

pepper, to taste

3 tablespoons water

Assembly

4 cups green leaf lettuce (320 g), chopped

1 cup cherry tomato (200 g), halved

¾ cup black beans (130 g)

½ cup corn (85 g)

⅓ cup fresh cilantro (15 g), chopped

⅓ cup red onion (50 g)

How To Prepare :

Cut the tempeh into a medium dice.

In a medium saucepan, heat a drizzle of olive oil over medium heat. Once the oil begins to shimmer, add the tempeh and cook for 6-8 minutes, until golden brown.

Add the soy sauce, garlic powder, chili powder, and cumin, stir, and cook for another 5 minutes, until all of the seasonings are well-distributed and the tempeh is browned. Remove the pan from the heat.

Make the avocado dressing: In a blender, combine the avocado, lime juice, olive oil, salt, and pepper and blend until smooth. Add the water 1 tablespoon at a time until your desired consistency is reached.

Arrange the lettuce, tomatoes, black beans, corn, cilantro, red onion, and tempeh in a large bowl and pour over the avocado dressing.

Enjoy!

Sweet Potato Chicken Stir-fry With Peanut Sauce

Ingredients

for 4 servings

2 tablespoons lime juice

2 tablespoons sesame oil

salt, to taste

pepper, to taste

1 lb boneless, skinless chicken breast (455 g), cut into 1-inch (2 1/2 cm) cubes

¼ cup creamy peanut butter (60 g)

1 tablespoon lime juice

1 tablespoon low sodium soy sauce

1 teaspoon rice wine vinegar

1 clove garlic, minced

1 teaspoon ginger, grated

½ teaspoon red pepper flakes

¼ cup water (60 mL)

1 small yellow bell pepper

1 small red bell pepper

1 small green bell pepper

1 medium sweet potato

2 cups broccoli floret (300 g)

½ tablespoon sesame oil

green onion, chopped, to serve

chopped peanut, to serve

How To Prepare :

In a small bowl, mix together peanut butter, lime juice, soy sauce, rice wine vinegar, garlic, ginger, red pepper flakes, and water until smooth. Set aside.

In a large bowl, mix lime juice, sesame oil, salt, and pepper.

Add cubed chicken to mixture and stir until completely coated.

Cover with plastic wrap and marinate in refrigerator for 30 minutes.

Heat a large skillet or saucepan over medium-high heat and add chicken. Cook for 4-6 minutes, or until no longer pink.

Once cooked through, remove chicken and transfer to a bowl.

Spiralize bell peppers and sweet potato into a large bowl.

Add sesame oil to the skillet. Once the oil is hot, add in the broccoli florets and cook for 2-3 minutes.

Add in the spiralized vegetables and cook for 2-3 minutes.

Add in the chicken and peanut sauce and stir to coat. NOTE: Add additional water if sauce is too thick to coat.

Reduce heat to medium low and cook for 3-4 minutes, until sweet potato noodles are al dente.

Top with green onions and chopped peanuts.

Enjoy!

Easy Chicken Cacciatore

Ingredients Needed

for 6 servings

4 boneless, skinless chicken breasts, cut in half, widthwise

salt, to taste

pepper, to taste

3 tablespoons oil, divided

1 lb portobello mushroom (455 g), diced

1 large white onion, diced

1 large red bell pepper, diced

4 cloves garlic, minced

2 teaspoons fresh rosemary, minced

14.5 oz diced tomato (410 g), 1 can

½ cup red wine (120 mL)

¾ cup low sodium chicken broth (180 mL), or vegetable broth

fresh basil, chopped, to serve

How To Prepare :

Season the chicken breasts on both sides with salt and pepper.

Heat 1 tablespoon of the oil in a large nonstick skillet over medium high heat.

Place 4 pieces of the chicken in the skillet and sear until until golden-brown, about 1-3 minutes on each side. Transfer the chicken to a plate and repeat searing with the remaining chicken pieces. Set aside.

Heat 1 tablespoon of oil in the empty skillet.

Add the mushrooms and stir occasionally until most of the moisture has evaporated from the pan, about 8 minutes.

Transfer the mushrooms to a plate and set aside.

Heat the remaining 1 tablespoon of oil in the pan.

Add the onions and bell peppers and season with salt and pepper. Stir occasionally until the onions and peppers have softened, about 2 minutes.

Add in the garlic and rosemary and stir until the garlic is fragrant.

Add in the tomatoes, red wine, and broth and stir until the sauce has thickened slightly.

Add the mushrooms and chicken back into the sauce and bring to a low simmer.

Cover and let cook until the chicken registers 165°F (74°C), about 5-8 minutes.

Serve topped with basil.

Enjoy!

Double Crunch Shrimp

Ingredients

for 4 servings

Shrimp

1 lb medium shrimp (455 g), peeled and deveined

salt, to taste

pepper, to taste

4 large eggs

1 ½ cups soda water (360 mL), cold

2 cups cake flour (200 g)

oil, for frying

The Everything Addison's Disease Diet Cookbook

3 cups panko bread crumbs (150 g)

Glaze

1 tablespoon oil

4 cloves garlic, minced

1 tablespoon ginger, minced

1 cup low-sodium soy sauce (240 mL)

2 tablespoons rice wine vinegar

⅓ cup light brown sugar (75 g)

1 pinch red pepper flakes

¼ cup water (60 mL)

1 tablespoon cornstarch

For Serving

white rice, cooked

scallion, thinly sliced

sesame seed

How To Prepare :

Pat the shrimp dry with paper towels, then transfer to a medium bowl and season with salt and pepper.

In a separate medium bowl, whisk the eggs and soda water until combined. Add the cake flour and gently whisk, making sure the batter is still clumpy. Do not overmix.

Heat the oil in a large pot until it reaches 350°F (180°C).

Add the panko bread crumbs to a shallow bowl.

Using a slotted spoon, dip the shrimp in the tempura batter, then toss in the panko, making sure to fully coat.

Fry the shrimp in the hot oil, 5-6 at a time, until golden brown, about 2-3 minutes. Transfer to a wire rack to drain.

Make the glaze: Heat the oil in a medium saucepan over medium-high heat. Add the garlic and ginger and cook until fragrant, about 30 seconds, stirring frequently.

Add the soy sauce, rice wine vinegar, brown sugar, and red pepper flakes. Stir until the mixture begins to simmer.

In a small bowl, combine the water and cornstarch. Add the cornstarch slurry to the saucepan and stir to combine. Cook until the glaze is reduced by half and looks thick and syrupy, about 5 minutes.

Transfer the shrimp to a large bowl and pour the glaze over. Toss the shrimp gently to coat with the glaze.

Serve the shrimp over rice and garnish with scallions.

Enjoy!

Sweet Potato "Fried" Rice

Ingredients

for 2 servings

2 medium-sized sweet potatoes, peeled and chopped

1 tablespoon cooking oil, of preference, or water

½ white onion, diced

2 large carrots, peeled and sliced

½ teaspoon salt

½ teaspoon pepper

½ cup vegetable broth (120 mL)

½ cup pea (75 g), cooked

2 eggs, scrambled

2 tablespoons low sodium soy sauce

green onion, chopped, for garnish

How To Prepare :

In a food processor, pulse the sweet potato chunks until they reach your desired "rice" consistency.

In a large skillet over medium heat, heat oil, then add onions and let cook until translucent.

Add sweet potato rice, carrots, salt, pepper, and vegetable broth and cook until the liquid has evaporated and the sweet potato is tender, stirring occasionally.

Add peas, eggs, and soy sauce, and combine, allowing it to heat through.

Garnish with green onions.

Enjoy!

Braised Chicken Thighs With Red Rice

Ingredients Needed

for 4 servings

Chicken

5 oz bone-in, skin-on chicken thighs (140 g)

½ teaspoon sea salt

¼ teaspoon freshly ground black pepper

1 tablespoon canola oil

1 cup yellow onion (150 g), minced

1 cup fresh tomato (200 g), diced

1 poblano chile, seeded and minced

3 cloves garlic, thinly sliced

¼ teaspoon hot smoked paprika

½ cup red wine vinegar (120 mL)

1 cup low sodium chicken stock (240 mL)

Red Rice

½ cup bacon (110 g), diced

½ medium red onion, diced

1 cup red bell pepper (100 g), seeded and diced

1 stalk celery, diced

½ jalapeño, red, seeded and minced

1 cup basmati rice (200 g)

1 cup chopped tomato (200 g), peeled and seeded, juices reserved

3 bay leaves, dried

sea salt, to taste

1 ½ cups low sodium chicken broth (360 mL)

How To Prepare :

Season the chicken thighs on both sides with the salt and pepper.

Heat the oil in a wide, heavy-bottomed pot with a lid over medium heat. When the oil is hot, add the chicken thighs, skin-side down and let cook without disturbing for 10 minutes. This will allow the skin to caramelize and develop a ton of flavor in the process. Turn the thighs over, cook for 1 minute more, then transfer to a plate.

Add the onion, tomatoes, poblano, garlic, and paprika to the pan. Cook for 5 minutes, until the vegetables are softened.

Carefully add the vinegar and stir to loosen any browned bits stuck to the bottom of the pot. Cook until the vinegar is reduced by half, 2-4 minutes, then pour in the stock.

Return the chicken to the pan, skin-side up. Cover and reduce the heat to low. Cook for 20 minutes, then remove lid and continue cooking until the internal temperature of the chicken thighs reaches 165°F (75°C).

Meanwhile, make the red rice: In a large pan, cook the slab bacon over medium heat until the fat renders and it begins to crisp, 5-8 minutes.

Add the onion, bell pepper, celery, and jalapeño and cook until softened, about 10 minutes.

Add the rice and stir until toasted, about 2 minutes.

Stir in the tomatoes, ½ cup (100 G) of the reserved tomato juice, bay leaves, and season with salt. 9. Add the chicken broth. Bring to a boil, then cover, reduce the heat to low, and simmer for 20 minutes, until the liquid is absorbed and the rice is tender.

Serve the chicken over the rice with some of the braising jus and vegetables ladled over.

Enjoy!

Tofu Scramble Breakfast Tacos

Ingredients

for 1 serving

1 tablespoon olive oil

⅓ block tofu

1 tablespoon low sodium soy sauce

1 tablespoon nutritional yeast

½ teaspoon turmeric

¾ teaspoon garlic powder

black pepper, to taste

1 cup spinach (40 g)

2 whole wheat tortillas

¼ avocado, sliced

½ red pepper, diced

hot sauce, optional

How To Prepare :

In a medium-sized sauté pan, add olive oil and tofu, and sauté until lightly browned.

Add in soy sauce, nutritional yeast, garlic powder, turmeric, black pepper, red pepper, and spinach, then sauté for 3-5 more minutes or until spinach is wilted.

Serve immediately on tortillas and top with avocado, and hot sauce.

Enjoy!

Vegetarian Baked Beans

Ingredients Needed

for 6 servings

2 tablespoons olive oil

1 small yellow onion, diced

3 cloves garlic, minced

1 teaspoon smoked paprika

1 teaspoon chili powder

1 teaspoon mustard powder

½ teaspoon salt

¼ teaspoon pepper

½ cup tomato paste (110 g)

¼ cup maple syrup (85 g)

3 tablespoons molasses

2 tablespoons low sodium soy sauce

3 tablespoons apple cider vinegar

1 teaspoon liquid smoke

¾ cup low sodium vegetable broth (180 mL)

15 oz great northern beans (425 g), 3 cans, drained and rinsed

How To Prepare :

Preheat the oven to 350°F (180°C).

In a large saucepan, heat the olive oil over medium heat. Once the oil begins to shimmer, add the onion and cook for 4-5 minutes, until semi-translucent.

Add the garlic and cook for another 2-3 minutes, until fragrant.

Add the paprika, chili powder, mustard powder, salt, and pepper and cook for 2 more minutes, until the spices are fragrant.

Add the tomato paste, maple syrup, molasses, soy sauce, apple cider vinegar, and liquid smoke and stir for 1-2 minutes, until well-combined.

Then, add the vegetable broth and stir until smooth, about 1 minute.

Add the beans and stir for 1-2 minutes, until evenly coated.

Cover and bake for 40 minutes, until the beans are bubbling. Uncover and bake for another 10 minutes, or until desired consistency is reached.

Stir well and serve.

Enjoy!

One-Pan Cider-Braised Pork Chops

Ingredients Needed

for 2 servings

Brine

4 cups water (960 mL)

2 dried bay leaves

4 cloves garlic, crushed

1 tablespoon black peppercorn

⅓ cup sea salt (80 g)

4 cups ice (560 g)

Pork Chops

2 bone-in pork chops, about 1-inch (2 -cm) thick

sea salt, to taste

pepper, to taste

1 tablespoon high-heat cooking oil, of choice, such as vegetable or peanut

2 shallots, diced

3 cups turnip (450 g), diced

1 tablespoon dijon mustard

1 tablespoon fresh sage, chopped

2 cups apple cider (480 mL)

1 cup reduced sodium chicken stock (240 mL)

1 bunch collard green, stemmed and toughly chopped

How To Prepare :

Make the brine: Combine the water, bay leaves, garlic, peppercorns, and salt in a medium pot over medium heat and stir until the salt is dissolved.

Remove the brine from heat and stir in the ice cubes.

Once the brine is cooled, add the pork chops to a glass dish and pour the brine over. Chill in the refrigerator for 1-10 hours.

Preheat the oven to 350°F (180°C).

Remove the pork chops from the brine and pat dry. Season generously with salt and pepper on both sides.

Heat the oil in a large cast iron or other ovenproof skillet over medium-high heat until nearly smoking. Add the pork chops and sear without disturbing until caramelized and browned on the first side, about 2 minutes, then flip and sear on the other side. Remove the pork chops from the pan and set aside.

Add the shallots to the pan and cook until they begin to soften and caramelize, stirring occasionally, about 2 minutes.

Add the turnips and season with salt, then spread in an even layer and let caramelize, stirring occasionally, about 5 minutes.

Stir in the mustard and sage. Cook for 1 minute more.

Pour in the apple cider and chicken stock. Bring to a boil, then reduce the heat to low-medium and simmer until the liquid is reduced by half, about 7 minutes.

Add the collard greens and stir to incorporate. Nestle the pork chops into the sauce, making sure that they are partly submerged.

Transfer the pan to the oven and cook for about 12 minutes, until the internal temperature of the pork chops reaches 135°F (57°C).

Remove from the oven and let rest for 10 minutes as the internal temperature continues to climb to 145°F (63°C).

Divide the pork chops, vegetables, and sauce between plates and serve.

Nutrition, Pork Chops without braising liquid: Calories: 470, Total fat: 27 grams, Sodium: 790 grams, Total carbs: 48 grams, Dietary fiber: 7 grams, Sugars: 6 grams, Protein: 48 grams Braising Liquid, ¼ cup (60 ml) serving - Calories: 20, Total fat: 0, Sodium: 48 grams, Total carbs: 5 grams, Dietary fiber: 0 grams, Sugars: 4 grams, Protein: 0 grams

Enjoy!

Bánh Mì Bowl With Crispy Tofu

Ingredients Needed

for 2 servings

16 oz extra firm tofu (455 g)

salt, to taste

pepper, to taste

½ cup low sodium soy sauce (120 mL)

¼ cup rice wine vinegar (60 mL)

1 teaspoon sesame oil

2 cloves garlic, minced

2 tablespoons ginger, finely grated

1 large cucumber

3 small carrots

To Serve

brown rice

fresh cilantro

green onion

red cabbage

radish, sliced

fresh mint

jalapeño, sliced

How To Prepare :

Preheat oven to 375°F (190°C).

Wrap tofu in an absorbent towel. Set cast-iron skillet or other heavy object on top for 15-20 minutes to remove extra moisture.

Unwrap tofu and cut into small cubes. Transfer to a baking sheet and season with a pinch of salt and pepper.

Bake for about 20 minutes, or until the tofu is firm to the touch and golden brown.

In a medium bowl, add soy sauce, vinegar, sesame oil, garlic, and ginger. Stir to combine.

Spiralize the cucumber and carrots into a large bowl.

Transfer veggies to a bowl and assemble with tofu, brown rice, cilantro, green onions, red cabbage, radishes, mint, jalapeños, and sauce.

Enjoy!

Tempeh Tacos

Ingredients Needed

for 2 servings

8 oz tempeh (825 g), 1 package

1 tablespoon olive oil

¼ yellow onion, diced

1 jalapeño, diced

¼ cup low sodium soy sauce (60 mL)

1 teaspoon cumin

2 teaspoons chili powder

2 teaspoons garlic powder

black pepper, to taste

tortilla, to serve

How To Prepare :

Add tempeh to food processor and pulse until a crumbly consistency is formed, making sure not to over-pulse.

Heat olive oil in pan over medium heat. Once the oil begins to shimmer, add the onion and sauté for 3 minutes.

Add jalapeño and sauté for 2 more minutes, or until onion is translucent.

Add ground tempeh and sauté for 4 minutes, or until tempeh is slightly golden.

Add soy sauce, cumin, chili powder, garlic powder and black pepper and continue to sauté for 3-5 more minutes or until desired consistency is reached.

Serve on warm tortillas with desired taco toppings.

Enjoy!

Stuffed Firecracker Chicken Rolls

Ingredients

for 4 servings

1 cup low sodium soy sauce

⅓ cup buffalo sauce (95 g)

4 cloves garlic, minced

⅓ cup honey (115 g)

4 tablespoons sweet chili sauce

1 ½ lb boneless, skinless chicken breast (680 g)

2 tablespoons olive oil

½ yellow onion, finely diced

2 bell peppers, finely diced

2 cups spinach (80 g)

How To Prepare :

In a shallow dish or large plastic bag, add the soy sauce, buffalo sauce, garlic, honey, and sweet chili sauce. After mixing, reserve half the marinade in a separate bowl for later.

On a cutting board, slice the chicken breasts horizontally, making sure not to slice all the way through. Cover chicken breast with parchment or plastic wrap and use a mallet to flatten the chicken, about ⅓ inch (8 mm) in thickness.

Place chicken breasts in the marinade and chill for about 2 hours or overnight.

Add 1 tablespoon of olive oil to a large pan over medium heat. Once hot, add garlic and cook until aromatic, about 30 seconds. Add the onion and bell peppers, and cook until soft.

Remove the chicken breast from the marinade and lay flat. Spoon a layer of the onion and the bell pepper mixture across the chicken breast, then add a layer of spinach.

Roll up chicken breast and secure with a toothpick, about 1½ inches (4 cm) apart. Cut the chicken breast in half.

Add 1 tablespoon of olive oil to a large pan over medium heat. Once hot, place chicken rolls inside the pan, cook until inside is no longer pink, about 6 minutes on each side. Remove from pan.

Add reserved marinade to the pan and cook until caramelized, about 3 minutes.

Serve drizzled in caramelized marinade.

Enjoy!

Teriyaki Chicken Cauliflower Rice Bowl

Ingredients Needed

for 1 serving

Teriyaki Sauce

1 tablespoon reduced sodium soy sauce

1 teaspoon maple syrup

1 clove garlic, minced

¼ teaspoon ginger, minced

¼ teaspoon cornstarch

¼ teaspoon freshly ground black pepper

1 cup broccoli floret (150 g)

2 cups cauliflower florets (300 g)

1 boneless, skinless chicken breast, sliced into 1/2 pieces

¼ teaspoon salt

¼ teaspoon ground black pepper

1 tablespoon olive oil

¼ cup green onion (35 g), plus 1 tbsp, sliced, divided

⅔ cup red cabbage (65 g), shredded

1 carrot, diced

1 teaspoon toasted white sesame seeds

How To Prepare :

In a bowl, add the soy sauce, maple syrup, garlic, ginger, cornstarch, and black pepper, and whisk until well combined.

Microwave broccoli on high for 1 minute.

Add the cauliflower to a food processor and pulse until it is the size of rice.

On a cutting board, season chicken breast with salt and pepper.

Heat olive oil in a large pan or wok over high heat. Once the oil begins to shimmer, add the chicken and cook until browned on both sides, about 2 minutes.

Add the teriyaki sauce and bring to a simmer.

Add ¼ cup (35 g) green onions, red cabbage, and carrots, and cook for 30 seconds.

Add cauliflower and cook, stirring constantly, for 1 minute. Add broccoli and remove from heat.

Top with sesame seeds and remaining green onions.

Enjoy!

Summertime Lentil Bolognese

Ingredients

for 8 servings

2 medium carrots, roughly chopped

1 large white onion, roughly chopped

3 celeries, roughly chopped

3 cloves garlic

1 cup raw walnut (100 g)

2 tablespoons olive oil

1 teaspoon dried basil

2 teaspoons dried oregano

1 teaspoon dried parsley

kosher salt, to taste

2 tablespoons tomato paste

2 ¾ cups low sodium vegetable broth (660 mL)

1 cup green lentil (200 g)

1 can diced tomato

½ cup red wine (120 mL)

noodle, for serving

6 medium zucchinis

2 tablespoons olive oil, plus more as needed

kosher salt, to taste

½ teaspoon red pepper flakes

3 cloves garlic, minced

6 medium zucchinis

2 tablespoons olive oil, plus more as needed

kosher salt, to taste

½ teaspoon red pepper flakes

3 cloves garlic, minced

How To Prepare :

In a food processor, combine the carrots, onion, celery, and garlic. Pulse until finely chopped, but not mushy. Transfer the vegetables to a bowl.

Add the walnuts to the food processor and pulse until they reach the consistency of ground meat.

Heat the olive oil in a large pot over medium-high heat. Add the vegetable mixture, basil, oregano, parsley, and salt. Cook for 25 minutes, stirring frequently, until caramelized and any excess moisture has evaporated. Add the tomato paste, stir to combine, and cook for 5 minutes.

Add the vegetable stock, lentils, ground walnuts, and tomatoes and season with salt. Reduce the heat to medium, cover, and simmer for 35 minutes, stirring occasionally, until the lentils are cooked through and walnuts have softened. Remove the lid and cook off any remaining liquid, stirring frequently, about 5 minutes.

Add the wine, stir, and reduce until there is no liquid at the bottom of the pot, about 10 minutes. Season with more salt to taste.

Trim the ends of the zucchini, then cut into noodles using a spiralizer or julienne peeler.

Add 2 tablespoons of olive oil, a pinch of salt, the red pepper flakes, and garlic to a large pan. Turn the heat to medium and cook for 2-3 minutes, until the garlic is fragrant.

Work in batches, add about 2-3 cups of zucchini noodles at a time to the pan. Season lightly with salt and cook for 45-60 seconds, tossing continuously with tongs, until warmed through. 9. Add more olive oil, 1 tablespoon at a time, if the pan looks dry.

Serve the zucchini noodles with the Bolognese.

Enjoy!

Vegan Instant Pot Quinoa Chili

Ingredients Needed

for 6 servings

1 tablespoon avocado oil

1 medium onion

1 cup zucchini (125 g), chopped

2 cups broccoli (300 g), chopped

1 cup celery (100 g), chopped

4 cloves garlic, finely minced

½ cup quinoa (100 g), rinsed, uncooked

1 can chili beans

½ teaspoon ground cumin

¼ teaspoon ground black pepper

2 teaspoons onion powder

2 teaspoons paprika

salt, to taste

red chili flake, optional

32 oz low sodium vegetable broth (7 L)

How To Prepare :

Set IP to Saute mode.

Heat avocado oil.

Add chopped garlic, vegetables, quinoa, chili beans and spices.

Saute for about 5 minutes, stirring occasionally.

Add vegetable stock and stir well.

Shut the IP lid. Change setting to Multigrain 9 minutes with valve in 'Sealing' position.

When IP beeps, you can either manually vent, or allow for natural release of steam. Carefully open the lid. Taste and adjust spices accordingly.

Korean-Style Bbq Beef Dinner Kit

Ingredients Needed

for 5 helpings

Tasty™ Korean-Style BBQ Beef Dinner Kit

1 lb sirloin steak (455 g), sliced in quarter-inch strips

1 medium red bell pepper, thinly sliced

1 tablespoon oil

1 ¾ cups water (420 mL)

½ teaspoon salt

Make It Special

4 stems green onion, diagonally cut

1 tablespoon sesame seeds

How To Prepare :

Add water, salt and rice to a 2-quart saucepan; stir. Bring to a boil.

Reduce heat to low. Cover; cook 22-24 minutes. Remove from heat and set aside.

Meanwhile, coat sliced beef with seasoning in shallow bowl or plastic bag.

Heat oil in 10-inch non-stick skillet over medium-high heat. Carefully add beef and peppers; cook 6 to 7 minutes, stirring occasionally, until sauce thickens.

Top rice with beef and peppers; drizzle with Korean BBQ Sauce. Sprinkle with optional toppings if desired. Enjoy!

Jazzy Shrimp And Grits

Ingredients Needed

for 4 servings

Shrimp

1 tablespoon McCormick® Jazzy Spice Blend

1 teaspoon kosher salt

½ teaspoon freshly ground black pepper

1 lb raw shrimp (455 g), peeled and deveined

Grits

4 cups water (960 mL), vegetable stock or chicken stock

1 cup stone ground corn grits (150 g)

1 cup shredded white cheddar (100 g)

1 tablespoon unsalted butter

1 teaspoon kosher salt

½ teaspoon pepper

Assembly

4 strips bacon, uncooked

3 cloves garlic, thinly sliced

¼ cup dry white wine (60 mL)

¼ cup chicken stock (60 mL), or vegetable stock

2 tablespoons fresh chives

How To Prepare :

Make the shrimp: In a medium bowl, mix together the Jazzy Spice Blend, salt, and pepper. Add the shrimp and toss to coat thoroughly. Cover with plastic wrap and marinate in the refrigerator for 1 hour.

Make the grits: In a large saucepan over high heat, bring the water or stock to a boil. Once boiling, whisk in the grits. Reduce the heat to low and simmer, whisking often, until the grits begin to thicken. If the grits are bubbling and spurting too much, cover the pot partially with a lid, but make sure not to cover fully. Continue whisking frequently until the grits are tender, about 1 hour. If the grits get too thick before they are fully cooked, add ¼ cup cooking liquid at a time. Once cooked, stir in the cheddar cheese, butter, salt, and pepper. Keep warm before serving.

While the grits are cooking, place the bacon strips in a cold medium skillet. Turn the heat to medium-low and cook the bacon until crispy, 2-3 minutes per side. Remove the bacon from the pan, leaving the bacon fat behind, and drain on paper towels. Once the bacon is cool, chop and reserve.

Add the garlic to the bacon fat in the pan and cook for 1-2 minutes over medium low heat until fragrant. Add the shrimp, white wine, and chicken stock to pan. Cook until the shrimp are pink and opaque, then remove from the pan.

Return chopped bacon to pan and cook for about a minute, until the liquid in the pan reduces slightly to make a sauce.

Spoon the grits into bowls and top with the shrimp. Spoon the bacon sauce over the shrimp and garnish with chives.

Enjoy!

Chicken Tikka Masala Dinner Kit

Ingredients Needed

for 5 helpings

Tasty™ Chicken Tikka Masala Dinner Kit

1 lb boneless, skinless chicken breast (455 g), cut in 1/2-inch cubes

1 medium onion, thinly sliced

2 tablespoons oil

1 ½ cups water (360 mL)

½ teaspoon salt

½ cup heavy cream (or milk) (120 mL)

Make It Special

3 tablespoons fresh cilantro, chopped

plain greek yogurt

How To Prepare :

Add water, salt and rice to a 2-quart saucepan; stir. Bring to a boil.

Reduce heat to low. Cover; cook 22-24 minutes. Remove from heat and set aside.

Meanwhile, coat chicken pieces with seasoning in shallow bowl or plastic bag.

Heat oil in 10-inch non-stick skillet over medium-high heat. Carefully add chicken and onions; cook 7 to 9 minutes, stirring frequently, until thoroughly cooked.

Reduce heat to low. Stir in Tikka Masala sauce and cream; cook 1-2 minutes until cooked through.

Serve chicken and onions with rice. Sprinkle with optional toppings if desired. Enjoy!

Herb Sea Salt-Rubbed Chicken Thighs

Ingredients Needed

for 4 servings

8 bone-in, skin-on chicken thighs

2 tablespoons herb sea salt

3 tablespoons olive oil

How To Prepare :

Preheat the oven to 425°F (220°C). Line a baking sheet with parchment paper and set a wire rack inside.

Pat the chicken thighs dry with a paper towel. Generously season the chicken on both sides with the herb salt, rubbing underneath the skin. Let sit for 15-20 minutes to draw out the moisture from the chicken skin, which will result in crispier chicken.

After resting, pat the chicken thighs dry once more to remove any excess moisture. Drizzle the olive oil under the skin and rub into the chicken.

Place the chicken thighs skin-side up on the wire rack. Bake for 30 minutes, until the skin is crispy and the internal temperature reaches 155-160°F (68-71°C).

Let the thighs rest for 15 minutes to bring the internal temperature to 165°F (75°C) and to let the juices settle.

Enjoy!

Fajita Pasta Bake

Ingredients Needed

for 6 servings

1 yellow bell pepper, seeded and sliced

1 green bell pepper, seeded and sliced

1 red bell pepper, seeded and sliced

2 ½ cups mushroom (185 g), sliced

1 medium yellow onion, diced

1 tablespoon chili powder

1 tablespoon paprika

1 tablespoon garlic powder

1 tablespoon cumin

1 teaspoon salt

1 teaspoon pepper

3 tablespoons olive oil

4 cups penne pasta (400 g), uncooked

1 ½ cups sour cream (345 g)

3 cups shredded pepper jack cheese (300 g)

fresh parsley, chopped. for garnish

How To Prepare :

Preheat the oven to 400°F (200°C).

In a nonstick baking dish, add the bell peppers, mushrooms, and onion.

In a small bowl, combine the chili powder, paprika, garlic powder, cumin, salt, and pepper.

Pour the olive oil and half of the spice mix over the vegetables and toss well to coat.

Bake the vegetables for about 30 minutes, stirring occasionally, until tender.

In a large pot of boiling water, cook the pasta according to the package instructions, until tender.

Drain the pasta, reserving about 1 cup (240 ml) of cooking water.

Return the drained pasta to the pot and add the roasted vegetables. Add the rest of the spice mix, the reserved pasta water, and the sour cream and mix to combine.

Transfer the pasta mixture to the baking dish used for roasting the vegetables and spread evenly. Sprinkle the cheese over the top.

Bake for about 15 minutes, until the cheese is golden brown.

Let cool for about 5 minutes, then serve. Garnish with parsley, if desired.

Enjoy!

Easily The Best Garlic Herb Roasted Potatoes

Ingredients Needed

for 5 servings

13 russet potatoes, cut into 1-inch (2 1/2 cm) pieces

1 teaspoon baking soda

1 teaspoon salt

¼ cup olive oil (60 mL)

2 tablespoons garlic, minced

2 tablespoons fresh rosemary, or fresh thyme, finely chopped

1 teaspoon black pepper

salt, to taste

pepper, to taste

1 small handful fresh parsley leaf, minced to garnish

How To Prepare :

Fill a large pot with water and boil. Add salt, baking soda, and potatoes, and stir.

Return to a boil, reduce to a simmer, and cook for 10 minutes after returning to a boil. A fork should easily pierce the potato pieces by the end. Drain and let sit one minute while moisture evaporates.

Combine olive oil, rosemary (or thyme), garlic, and a few grinds of black pepper in a small saucepan and heat over medium heat. Stir constantly until garlic just begins to turn golden, about 2-3 minutes.

Immediately strain oil through a fine-mesh strainer over the potatoes. Add salt and pepper to taste, and mix.

Shake the pot that the potatoes are in so that they slam against all sides of the pot, this will loosen the outer layer of the potatoes to form a mashed layer around each potato piece.

Preheat oven to 425°F (220°C).

Transfer potatoes to a large rimmed baking sheet and separate them, spreading them out evenly.

Transfer to oven and roast, without moving, for 30-35 minutes.

Using a thin, flexible metal spatula flip potatoes. Continue roasting until potatoes are deep brown and crisp all over, turning and shaking them a few times during cooking, 30 to 40 minutes longer.

Transfer potatoes to a large bowl and add the garlic-rosemary mixture (optional) and minced parsley. Toss to coat and season with more salt and pepper to taste. Serve immediately.

Enjoy!

Spinach Artichoke Penne Pasta

Ingredients Needed

for 3 servings

2 tablespoons olive oil

5 oz spinach (140 g)

1 cup artichoke heart (170 g), drained

16 oz cream cheese (455 g), softened

1 tablespoon garlic powder

1 teaspoon salt

1 teaspoon pepper

2 cups milk (470 mL)

4 cups penne pasta (400 g), cooked

How To Prepare :

Heat oil in a large pot over medium heat. Add spinach, cooking until wilted, then add artichoke hearts, cooking for 1 minute.

Add cream cheese until melted, stirring until there are no lumps.

Sprinkle in garlic powder, salt, pepper, and milk, stirring until smooth.

Add pasta and mix until pasta is evenly coated.

Nutrition Calories: 1589 Fat: 71 grams Carbs: 190 grams Fiber: 11 grams Sugars: 20 grams Protein: 46 grams

Enjoy!

Garlic Chicken Primavera

Ingredients Needed

for 4 servings

2 tablespoons olive oil

3 cloves garlic, chopped

2 chicken breasts, thinly sliced

2 cups asparagus (250 g), chopped

1 cup cherry tomato (200 g), halved

1 cup carrot (120 g), sliced

1 teaspoon pepper

1 teaspoon salt

4 cups penne pasta (400 g)

1 cup parmesan cheese (110 g)

How To Prepare :

Heat oil in a large pot over high heat. Cook garlic and chicken until no pink is showing.

Add asparagus, tomatoes, carrots, salt, and pepper, cooking for about 2 minutes.

Add pasta and parmesan, stirring until cheese is melted and evenly distributed.

Serve.

Enjoy!

Chicken Fajita Quesadilla

Ingredients Needed

for 2 quesadillas

½ lb chicken breast (225 g), cut into thin strips

½ teaspoon salt

½ teaspoon pepper

½ tablespoon chili powder

½ teaspoon cumin

¼ teaspoon cayenne

¼ teaspoon garlic powder

½ cup bell pepper (50 g), green, red, or yellow peppers, julienned

½ cup white onion (75 g), julienned

2 large flour tortillas

1 cup shredded cheddar cheese (100 g), double for 2 quesadillas

1 cup shredded monterey jack cheese (100 g), double for 2 quesadillas

Garnish

fresh cilantro

guacamole

sour cream

pico de gallo, or salsa

How To Prepare :

In a large skillet, coat chicken with salt, pepper, chili powder, cumin, cayenne, and garlic powder. Cook 5-7 minutes.

Add the peppers and onions and cook for 5-7 minutes, or until they are soft. Remove chicken, onions and peppers from the pan and set aside.

Place the tortilla in the skillet and add a layer of cheese on half of the tortilla.

Add cooked chicken, peppers and onions. Top with more cheese and fold the tortilla in half.

Cook for 6 minutes over medium heat, flipping half way.

Garnish with fresh cilantro and serve with pico de gallo, guacamole, and sour cream on the side.

Enjoy!

Chinese Chicken Curry

Ingredients Needed

for 2 servings

3 tablespoons oil

3 cups chicken (400 g)

1 teaspoon salt

1 teaspoon pepper

1 ⅓ cups onion (200 g), chopped

¾ cup carrot (100 g), chopped

1 cup potato (200 g), chopped

4 ¼ cups water (1 L)

⅔ cup peas (100 g)

⅔ cup curry paste (150 g)

How To Prepare :

Heat up 2 tablespoons of oil on low to medium heat.

Sear the chicken until the outside turns golden brown. Season with salt and pepper.

Take out the chicken, make sure you don't clean the pot or you'd wipe away some deliciousness!

Add another tablespoon of oil, fry the onions, carrots, and potatoes until soften.

Add the chicken back in with the water. Bring to a boil then simmer for 10 minutes with the lid on.

Add in the peas and curry paste, stir well.

Serve with rice.

Enjoy!

Sun-Dried Tomato & Spinach Tuna Pasta

Ingredients Needed

for 2 servings

1 tablespoon olive oil

1 tablespoon garlic, minced

½ cup sundried tomato (25 g)

1 lemon, juiced

10 oz tuna (285 g), canned, drained

salt, to taste

pepper, to taste

2 cups whole wheat pasta (200 g), cooked according to package instructions

2 cups fresh spinach (80 g)

How To Prepare :

Heat the olive oil in a large skillet over medium-high heat. Add the garlic and cook for about 30 seconds, until fragrant.

Add the sun-dried tomatoes and lemon juice and cook for 1-2 minutes, until fragrant.

Add the tuna, salt, and pepper, and mix until thoroughly combined.

Add the pasta and spinach and cook for about 1 minute, until spinach starts to wilt.

Remove the pasta from the heat and serve.

Enjoy!

Chicken Teriyaki Chow Mein

Ingredients

for 6 servings

1 lb chicken breast (455 g), cubed

salt, to taste

pepper, to taste

½ cup teriyaki sauce (120 mL), divided

4 tablespoons cooking oil, divided

6 oz chow mein noodle (180 g), hong kong style pan fried noodles, par cooked according to package instructions

¾ cup onion (11520 g), sliced

½ cup carrot (60 g), julienned

1 cup broccoli floret (150 g)

1 cup cabbage (100 g)

sesame seed, for garnish

How To Prepare :

In a medium bowl, season the cubed chicken with salt and pepper. Add ¼ cup (of 60 ml) teriyaki sauce and mix until the chicken is well-coated. Cover with plastic wrap and marinate in the refrigerator for 30 minutes to 1 hour.

In a wok or deep skillet over medium-high heat, heat 2 tablespoons of cooking oil, then add the par-cooked noodles. Cook for 1-2 minutes, allowing the noodles to crisp, then flip and cook for another 1-2 minutes. Transfer to a plate and set aside.

In the same wok, heat 1 tablespoon of cooking oil, then add the chicken. Cook for 3-4 minutes, until browned on one side, then stir and cook for another 3-4 minutes, until fully cooked through. Set the chicken aside.

In the same wok, add 1 tablespoon of oil, the onion, and carrot. Cook for 2-3 minutes, or until the onions are translucent. Add the broccoli and cabbage. Stir and cook for 1-2 minutes, then season with salt and pepper and cook for 3 minutes more, until the vegetables are soft.

Add the cooked chicken and crispy noodles back to the wok, along with the remaining ¼ cup (60 ml) teriyaki sauce. Toss well and cook for 2-3 minutes, until everything is well-combined. Garnish with sesame seeds.

Enjoy!

CHAPTER 6
ADDISON DISEASE FRIENDLY SOUP AND STEW RECIPES

Buffalo Cauliflower Nachos

Ingredients Needed

for 6 servings

1 head cauliflower, cut into florets

3 tablespoons olive oil

1 tablespoon smoked paprika

fine sea salt, to taste

freshly ground black pepper, to taste

2 tablespoons hot sauce

2 tablespoons siracha

1 tablespoon butter, melted

1 lime, juiced

8 cups tortilla chips (800 g)

1 cup monterey jack cheese (100 g), grated

1 cup cheddar cheese (100 g), grated

1 avocado, chopped

3 radishes, thinly sliced

2 celery stems, thinly sliced

sour cream, to serve

fresh cilantro, chopped, to serve

How To Prepare :

Preheat oven to 400°F (200°C).

On a large baking sheet, toss together the cauliflower florets, olive oil, paprika, salt, and pepper. Roast until tender, 20-25 minutes.

In a large bowl, whisk together the hot sauce, sriracha, melted butter, and lime juice.

Add the roasted cauliflower to the bowl and mix to coat.

Scatter the tortilla chips over the baking sheet. Top with the cauliflower, Monterey Jack cheese, and cheddar cheese.

Return the baking sheet to the oven and bake until cheese is melted and bubbling, about 5 minutes.

Top with avocado, radishes, celery, sour cream, and cilantro. Serve warm.

Enjoy!

Family Borscht Recipe By Andrew

Ingredients Needed

for 10 servings

1 cup mixed dried mushroom (75 g)

1 ½ lb small beet (680 g)

2 tablespoons whole black peppercorn

2 whole allspice berries

12 garlics, peeled

2 bay leaves

1 tablespoon canola oil

2 leeks, rinsed well and thinly sliced

1 small yellow onion, diced

1 stalk celery, diced

kosher salt, to taste

4 qt water (4 L)

1 large idaho potato, peeled and cubed

2 carrots, diced

15 oz stewed tomato (425 g)

8 oz tomato sauce (225 g)

16 oz pickled beet (455 g), drained and julienned

fresh dill, chopped, to taste

1 loaf dark rye bread, for serving, optional

sour cream, for serving, optional

How To Prepare :

Place the dried mushrooms in a medium bowl and pour in enough water to cover. Let soak for 20-30 minutes, or until the mushrooms are soft and plumped. Working over the bowl, squeeze any excess water from the mushrooms. Reserve the soaking liquid, and chop the mushrooms into bite-size pieces. Set aside.

Trim and peel the beets, then grate on the large holes of a box grater. You should have about 8 cups grated beets. Set aside.

Make a bouquet garni: Place the peppercorns, allspice, garlic, and bay leaves on a double-layer square of cheesecloth. Tie the ends of the cheesecloth around the spices and set aside.

In a large pot, heat the canola oil over medium heat. Add the leeks, onion, and celery. Season with salt and cook until the vegetables have softened, 5-8 minutes.

Add the water, grated beets, chopped mushrooms and reserved soaking liquid, and the bouquet garni. Bring to a boil then lower the heat and simmer for 20-30 minutes, or until the beets are tender.

Add the potato and season with a pinch of salt. Cook until potatoes are tender, 10-15 minutes, then add the carrots and cook until tender, 10 minutes more.

Add the tomatoes, tomato sauce, and pickled beets. Cook for another 10 minutes, or until all of the vegetables are tender. Stir in the dill, then remove the pot from the heat.

Ladle the borscht into bowls. Garnish with dill and serve with rye bread and sour cream, if using.

Enjoy!

Chicken And Kale Stew

Ingredients Needed

for 6 servings

3 fresh bay leaves

2 sprigs fresh rosemary

4 sprigs fresh thyme

1 large sprig fresh sage

1 lb chicken thighs (455 g), cut into 1 1/2 in (3 cm) pieces

3 ½ teaspoons kosher salt, divided

2 tablespoons olive oil, divided

2 tablespoons unsalted butter

1 white onion, thinly sliced

3 medium carrots, cut into 1/2 (1 1/4 cm) in rounds

3 large cloves garlic, smashed

¼ teaspoon red pepper flakes, optional, plus more for serving

¼ cup all-purpose flour (30 g)

½ cup dry white wine (120 mL), such as sauvignon blanc

6 cups low sodium chicken stock (15 g)

2 ½ cups small red potato (560 g), quartered

1 bunch lacinato kale, stemmed and torn into 2 in (5 cm) pieces

½ teaspoon freshly ground black pepper, plus more to taste

freshly grated parmesan cheese, for serving

How To Prepare :

Make the bouquet garni: Stack the bay leaves, rosemary, thyme, and sage on top of one another.

Tie a 3-inch (7 cm) length of butcher's twine around the center of herbs and secure with a knot. Set aside.

Season the chicken all over with about 1 teaspoon salt.

In a large, heavy-bottomed pot, heat 2 tablespoons of olive oil over medium-high heat until shimmering. Add the chicken and cook for 1–2 minutes on one side, until golden brown and crispy. Flip and cook for another 1–2 minutes, until golden brown. Remove the chicken from the pot and set aside.

Reduce the heat to medium and add the remaining tablespoon of oil if the pot looks dry. Melt the butter until just bubbling. Add the onion and carrots and season with ½ teaspoon salt. Cook for 2–3 minutes, stirring occasionally, until the onion is translucent and carrot is beginning to soften. Stir in the garlic and red pepper flakes, if using. Add the flour and cook for 2–3 minutes, until the vegetables are well-coated and the flour is lightly toasted, stirring occasionally to prevent burning.

Deglaze the pan with the wine, scraping up any browned bits on the bottom of the pan.

Add the chicken stock, bouquet garni, 2–3 teaspoons of salt, and the potatoes. Increase the heat to medium-high and bring to a boil. Once boiling, reduce the heat to medium-low, cover, and simmer for 20–25 minutes, until the potatoes are tender.

Return the chicken to the pot, along with the kale. Season the stew with more salt to taste and the black pepper. Cook until the chicken is warmed through and the kale is just wilted and tender, and the chicken is cooked through, about 2–3 minutes.

Ladle the stew into bowls and top with freshly grated Parmesan cheese and more red pepper flakes. Serve warm.

Enjoy!

Immunity Boosting Green Soup

Ingredients Needed

for 8 servings

2 tablespoons olive oil

8 cloves garlic, minced

fresh ginger, peeled and sliced 3 inches (7cm)

4 scallions, chopped

3 tablespoons fresh oregano leaf

1 cup fresh parsley (35 g), plus more for serving

¼ teaspoon cayenne

1 teaspoon ground turmeric

½ teaspoon black pepper

2 tablespoons low sodium soy sauce

4 cups broccoli florets (600 g), tough stems trimmed

6 cups chicken stock (1.5 L), or vegetable stock

4 cups swiss chard (145 g), loosely packed, thick stems trimmed, roughly chopped

1 lb baby spinach (455 g)

1 avocado, ripe, diced

¼ cup lemon juice (60 mL)

kosher salt, to taste

pumpkin seed, toasted, for garnish

How To Prepare :

Heat the olive oil in a large pot over medium heat. Add the garlic, ginger, and scallions. Sauté for about 3 minutes, until very fragrant but not browned.

Add the oregano, parsley, cayenne, turmeric, black pepper, and soy sauce. Cook for 2 minutes, until the herbs begin to wilt.

Add the broccoli and cook until bright green and beginning to release some moisture, about 5 minutes.

Add the chicken stock. Cover, reduce the heat to low, and simmer for about 10 minutes, until the broccoli starts to soften.

Add the Swiss chard and stir until wilted, about 30 seconds. Add the baby spinach, a few handfuls at a time. Cook until just wilted and stir to incorporate into the soup before adding more. Once the spinach is wilted and the broccoli stems can be easily pierced with a fork, remove the soup from the heat. It is important not to overcook the greens, as they will begin to lose their vibrant color and nutrients.

Cool the soup for 15 minutes, until it can be safely transferred to a high-speed blender, if using. With a standing blender or immersion blender, puree the soup briefly to combine, then add the avocado, lemon juice, and salt and blend until creamy, with no lumps remaining.

Enjoy the soup hot or cold, garnished with toasted pumpkin seeds and parsley, if desired.

Enjoy!

Eggplant Potato Tomato Stew

Ingredients Needed

for 5 servings

4 medium yukon potatoes

2 medium eggplants, chopped

2 red bell peppers, seeded and chopped

5 tablespoons olive oil, divided

1 teaspoon salt, plus more to taste, divided

¾ teaspoon pepper, plus more to taste, divided

1 medium yellow onion, diced

1 tablespoon tomato paste

3 cloves garlic, minced

1 teaspoon smoked paprika

15 oz chickpeas (425 g), 1 can, drained and rinsed

3 medium beefsteak tomatoes, diced

1 ½ cups low sodium vegetable broth (360 mL)

fresh parsley, for serving

How To Prepare :

Preheat the oven to 400°F (200°C).

With a sharp knife, score a ring around each potato, just deep enough to break the skin. Place the potatoes in a medium pot of cold water. Bring to a boil and cook for about 8 minutes, until about halfway cooked.

Drain the potatoes, and rinse with cold water. Peel off the skin.

Cut the potatoes into ½-inch (1 cm) pieces and set aside.

Divide the eggplant and bell peppers between 2 baking sheets and spread in an even layer. Drizzle with 4 tablespoons of olive oil, and season with salt and pepper to taste. Toss with your hands to coat.

Bake for 25 minutes, flipping halfway through.

Heat the remaining tablespoon of olive oil in a large pot over medium heat. Once the oil begins to shimmer, add the onion and cook for 3-4 minutes, until semi-translucent.

Add the tomato paste and stir until well distributed, then add the garlic, paprika, 1 teaspoon salt, and ¾ teaspoon pepper, and cook for another 2-3 minutes, until fragrant.

Add the potatoes, chickpeas, and tomatoes, and stir to incorporate.

Stir in the vegetable broth and cover. Reduce the heat to low and cook for 20 minutes, until the potatoes are tender.

Add the roasted eggplant and bell pepper, and stir to combine. Cook for another 5-10 minutes, until the tomatoes have mostly broken down.

Ladle into bowls, garnish with parsley, and serve. Or, transfer the stew to resealable containers and store in the fridge for up to 5 days or freezer for up to 3 months.

Enjoy!

Hearty Buffalo Chicken Soup

Ingredients Needed

for 4 servings

1 stick unsalted butter

2 cups large yellow onion (300 g), diced

3 carrots, diced

3 stalks celery, diced

½ teaspoon kosher salt

1 cup buffalo sauce (260 g)

4 cups low sodium chicken broth (960 mL)

½ cup heavy cream (120 mL)

3 cups rotisserie chicken (375 g), shredded

4 small bread bowls, for serving

½ cup crumbled blue cheese (55 g), for garnish

2 scallions, thinly sliced, for garnish

How To Prepare :

Melt the butter in a large stock pot over medium heat. Add the onion, carrots, and celery. Cook, stirring occasionally, until the onions are translucent, about 3 minutes. Season with the salt.

Add the buffalo sauce and cook until the liquid is reduced and thickened, about 8 minutes.

Add the chicken stock and bring the soup to a boil. Reduce the heat to medium-low and simmer until thickened, about 30 minutes. Remove the pot from the heat and stir in the heavy cream and shredded chicken.

Ladle the soup into the bread bowls and garnish with the crumbled blue cheese and scallions. Serve warm.

Enjoy!

Hearty White Bean Stew

Ingredients

for 6 servings

1 medium leek

1 tablespoon olive oil

5 oz pancetta (140 g)

2 cups carrot (220 g), diced

3 stalks celery stalk, sliced

8 oz cremini mushroom (225 g), sliced

3 cloves garlic, minced

kosher salt, to taste

4 sprigs fresh thyme sprigs

14.5 oz diced tomato (410 g)

4 cups great northern beans (680 g), cooked or canned

6 cups low sodium vegetable broth (1.4 L)

parmesan cheese, freshly grated, for serving

bread, crusty, for serving

How To Prepare :

Trim the root end and the tough, dark green top of the leek and remove any thick outer layers. Cut the leek in half lengthwise, then slice into ¼-inch (6-mm) thick half moons.

Transfer to a bowl of water and shake around with your fingers to loosen any dirt or grit. Let the leeks sit in the water for a couple minutes to let any grit to sink to the bottom of the bowl. Carefully remove the cleaned leeks from the bowl, leaving the dirty water behind.

Heat the olive oil in a large, heavy-bottomed pot over medium heat. Add the pancetta and cook until crispy and most of the fat has rendered, about 8 minutes.

Add the leeks, carrots, celery, mushrooms, and garlic. Season with salt. Cook for 5-6 minutes, until the vegetables have released their juices and begin to soften.

Add the thyme leaves, tomatoes, beans, and vegetable stock. Stir to combine, then bring to a boil, cover, and cook, stirring occasionally, for 20 minutes until slightly reduced and hot throughout. Season with more salt, to taste.

Ladle into bowls and top with freshly grated Parmesan cheese. Serve with crusty bread.

Enjoy!

CHAPTER 7
ADDISON DISEASE FRIENDLY SALAD RECIPES

Mushroom And Garlic Quinoa Salad

Ingredients

for 2 servings

2 tablespoons olive oil

1 lb mushroom (455 g)

1 tablespoon dried thyme

1 teaspoon salt

3 cloves garlic, minced

1 ½ cups vegetable stock (355 mL)

1 cup water (235 mL)

1 cup quinoa (170 g)

cheese, of choice, grated to serve

How To Prepare :

In a medium-sized frying pan combine oil, mushrooms, thyme, and salt, then mix. Allow to cook about 5 minutes.

Add the garlic, cook for 6-8 more minutes minutes until mushrooms are sufficiently cooked through and beginning to crisp up. Set mushroom mixture aside.

Combine vegetable stock and water in pan, bring to a boil, then add quinoa and cover. Simmer for 12-15 minutes.

Add mushroom mixture to quinoa and garnish with grated cheese of your choice (optional).

Enjoy!

Tortilla Bowl Southwestern Salad

Ingredients Needed

for 4 servings

4 teaspoons vegetable oil

4 large flour tortillas

2 romaine lettuce hearts

2 tomatoes

½ red onion

2 avocados

1 cup corn (175 g), canned, rinsed and drained

1 cup black beans (170 g), canned, rinsed and drained

¼ cup olive oil (60 mL)

¼ cup lime juice (60 mL)

1 clove garlic, minced

⅛ teaspoon cumin

½ teaspoon red pepper flakes

3 tablespoons fresh cilantro, chopped

½ teaspoon salt

½ teaspoon pepper

How To Prepare :

Preheat the oven to 350°F (180°C).

Pour the vegetable oil (1 teaspoon per bowl) into medium (1.2 quart) oven-proof bowls and rub around to coat the surface. Press each tortilla into a greased bowl.

Bake for about 10 minutes, until golden brown. Let the tortilla bowls cool.

Make 3 cuts lengthwise on each of the romaine hearts, remove the stems, and chop into smaller pieces. Rinse, drain, and place in a large salad bowl.

Dice the tomatoes and add them to the bowl with the romaine.

Dice the onion and add it to the salad.

Cut the avocados in half, remove the pits, and dice. Add to the salad.

Add the corn and black beans.

In a small bowl or liquid measuring cup, combine the olive oil, lime juice, garlic, cumin, red pepper flakes, cilantro, salt, and pepper. Mix well.

Pour the dressing over the salad and toss well.

Fill each tortilla bowl with the salad.

Enjoy!

Roasted Veggie Quinoa Salad

Ingredients

for 4 servings

½ cup zucchini (75 g), cubed

½ cup sweet potato (100 g), cubed

1 cup cherry tomato (200 g), halved

½ red onion, diced

½ cup corn (85 g), fresh or canned

½ lemon, for juice

4 tablespoons olive oil, divided

1 teaspoon garlic salt, to taste

pepper, to taste

4 cups quinoa (680 g), cooked

1 tablespoon apple cider vinegar

¼ cup fresh parsley (10 g), chopped

How To Prepare :

Preheat the oven to 350°F (180°C). Line a baking sheet with parchment paper.

Add the zucchini, sweet potato, tomatoes, onion, and corn to the baking sheet.

Drizzle with the lemon juice and 2 tablespoons of olive oil, then season with garlic salt and pepper. Toss to coat evenly, keeping the vegetables separate on the pan.

Roast for 15-20 minutes, or until fork tender.

Transfer the roasted vegetables to a large bowl, and add the quinoa. Toss well.

In a small bowl, mix together the remaining 2 tablespoons of olive oil and apple cider vinegar. Pour over the veggies and quinoa, and toss to coat.

Garnish with parsley.

Enjoy!

Tuna Salad With Roasted Veggies

Ingredients Needed

for 2 servings

1 cup green beans (360 g), trimmed

2 cups baby potato (500 g), halved

1 lemon, sliced

1 tablespoon olive oil, divided

½ teaspoon salt, plus more to taste

½ teaspoon pepper, plus more to tate

½ teaspoon paprika

1 tablespoon fresh rosemary, minced

1 tablespoon fresh thyme, minced

3 cloves garlic, minced

1 red bell pepper, halved and seeded

mixed greens salad

hard-boiled egg, optional

2 tablespoons balsamic vinaigrette, optional

Tuna salad

10 oz tuna (285 g), canned, drained

1 stalk celery, diced

¼ cup greek yogurt (60 g)

salt, to taste

pepper, to taste

1 teaspoon fresh parsley

How To Prepare :

Preheat the oven to 375°F (190°C).

On a baking sheet lined with parchment paper, add the green beans, potatoes, and lemon.

Drizzle the vegetables with 2 teaspoons of olive oil and season with salt, pepper, paprika, rosemary, thyme, and garlic. Mix until evenly coated.

Add the bell pepper halves to the center of the baking sheet and drizzle with the remaining teaspoon of olive oil, ½ teaspoon of salt, and ½ teaspoon of pepper.

Roast for 20 minutes until vegetables are golden brown. Let cool.

Make the tuna salad: combine the tuna, celery, Greek yogurt, salt, pepper, and parsley in a medium bowl.

Add a large handful of greens to 2 bowls. Divide the roasted vegetables and bell pepper halves between the bowls. Add a hard-boiled egg, if desired. Scoop the tuna salad into the bell peppers.

Serve with a balsamic vinaigrette, if desired.

Enjoy!

Roasted Cauliflower Salad

Ingredients Needed

for 4 servings

1 medium head cauliflower, cut into florets

3 large carrots, cut into 1 inch (2.5 cm) pieces

1 tablespoon ground cumin

2 teaspoons paprika

kosher salt, to taste

black pepper, to taste

2 tablespoons olive oil

¼ medium red onion, thinly sliced

1 cup fresh italian parsley (35 g), roughly chopped

Dressing

¼ cup tahini (60 mL)

1 clove garlic, grated

2 tablespoons lemon juice

¼ cup water (60 mL)

¼ cup olive oil (60 mL)

kosher salt, to taste

pepper, to taste

How To Prepare :

Preheat the oven to 425°F (220°C). Line a baking sheet with parchment paper.

In a large bowl, combine the cauliflower, carrots, cumin, paprika, salt, pepper and olive oil. Toss until well-coated.

Spread the vegetables on the baking sheet in a single layer and roast for 20-25 minutes, until the carrots are tender.

Make the dressing: In a medium bowl, whisk together the tahini, garlic, lemon juice, and water. While whisking, slowly drizzle in the olive oil until the dressing is emulsified. Season with salt and pepper.

In a large bowl, mix together the onion and parsley. Add the roasted cauliflower and carrots, and toss well.

Drizzle the salad with the dressing, then serve.

Enjoy!

Sweet Potato And Chickpea Salad

Ingredients Needed

for 4 servings

2 large sweet potatoes, or 3 small, scrubbed

½ medium red onion

15 oz chickpeas (425 g), 1 can, rinsed and drained

½ cup olive oil (120 mL)

¼ cup lemon juice (60 mL)

2 tablespoons garlic, minced

1 teaspoon ground cumin

1 teaspoon paprika

¼ teaspoon cinnamon

¼ teaspoon cayenne

salt, to taste

pepper, to taste

3 oz mixed greens (85 g)

¼ cup fresh parsley (10 g), chopped

¼ cup fresh cilantro (10 g), chopped

dried cranberry, for garnish, optional

How To Prepare :

Preheat the oven to 425°F (220°C).

Cut the sweet potatoes in small cubes and transfer on one half of a non-stick baking sheet.

Peel and slice the onion and set aside.

Add the chickpeas to the other half of the baking sheet.

In a liquid measuring cup with a pour spout, combine the olive oil, lemon juice, garlic, cumin, paprika, cinnamon, cayenne, salt, and pepper and mix well.

Pour half of the dressing over the sweet potatoes and chickpeas and mix with your hands until well-coated. Keep the chickpeas and sweet potatoes separated as much as possible.

Scoot the chickpeas toward the sweet potatoes and add the onions to the baking sheet. Make sure everything is spread out evenly.

Bake for 30 minutes, until the sweet potatoes are tender. Use tongs to stir halfway through. Let cool for 20 minutes.

Place the greens in a large bowl. Top with the roasted chickpeas, sweet potatoes, and onion.

Add the parsley, cilantro, and remaining dressing and toss to combine.

Top with dried cranberries, if using.

Enjoy!

Three Bean Salad

Ingredients

for 5 servings

½ red onion

½ large english cucumber

½ cup fresh parsley

15 oz chickpeas (425 g), 1 can, drained and rinsed

15 oz kidney bean (425 g), 1 can, drained and rinsed

15 oz cannellini bean (425 g), 1 can, drained and rinsed

¼ cup olive oil (60 mL)

¼ cup red wine vinegar (60 mL)

½ teaspoon dried oregano

½ teaspoon salt

¼ teaspoon pepper

How To Prepare :

Thinly slice the red onion and add to a large bowl.

Quarter the cucumber, remove the seeds and dice, then add to the bowl with the red onion.

Use a fork to remove the leaves from the parsley, then finely chop and add to the bowl.

Add the chickpeas, kidney beans, and cannellini beans to the bowl.

In a liquid measuring cup or small bowl, combine the olive oil, red wine vinegar, oregano, salt, and pepper, and whisk together.

Pour the dressing over the salad and mix well until evenly distributed.

Enjoy!

Chicken, Cranberry, And Pear Spinach Salad

Ingredients Needed

for 1 serving

Apple Cider Vinaigrette

3 tablespoons olive oil

2 tablespoons apple cider vinegar

1 teaspoon honey

½ teaspoon dijon mustard

¼ teaspoon salt

1 pinch ground black pepper

Salad

1 boneless, skinless chicken breast, sliced into 1/2-inch (1 cm) pieces

½ teaspoon salt

¼ teaspoon ground black pepper

¼ teaspoon paprika

1 tablespoon olive oil

1 pear, sliced

2 cups baby spinach (80 g)

1 tablespoon dried cranberry

2 tablespoons toasted unsalted walnut, chopped

How To Prepare :

Add the olive oil, apple cider vinegar, honey, Dijon mustard, salt, and pepper together in a small bowl. Set aside.

On a cutting board, season the chicken with salt, pepper, and paprika.

Heat olive oil in a pan over medium heat. Once the oil begins to shimmer, add the chicken and cook until browned on all sides, about 4 minutes.

In a large bowl, add the sliced pear, spinach, cranberries, walnuts, and cooked chicken, and dress with the vinaigrette.

Enjoy!

Charred Summer Vegetable Salad

Ingredients Needed

for 4 servings

Charred Vegetable Salad

2 zucchinis, halved lengthwise and cut into 1-inch (2 cm) half moons

1 yellow bell pepper, seeded and cut into 1-inch (2 cm) pieces

1 red onion, quartered, root left intact

2 ears corn, husked

¼ cup olive oil (60 mL)

1 teaspoon kosher salt

½ teaspoon freshly ground black pepper

3 cups baby arugula (120 g)

1 cup cherry tomato (200 g), halved

½ cup crumbled goat cheese (55 g)

Lemon Basil Dressing

½ cup extra virgin olive oil (120 mL)

¼ cup fresh lemon juice (60 mL)

½ cup fresh basil leaves (20 g)

1 tablespoon honey

¼ teaspoon ground black pepper

½ teaspoon kosher salt

1 small clove garlic, peeled

How To Prepare :

Char the vegetables: Arrange an oven rack in the top third of the oven. Turn the oven to high broil.

On a rimmed baking sheet, arrange the zucchini, bell pepper, red onion, and corn. Drizzle with the olive oil and season with the salt and pepper.

Broil the vegetables for 8–10 minutes, until softened and nicely charred in spots. Remove from the oven and let vegetables cool enough to handle, about 20 minutes.

While the vegetables cool, make the dressing: In a blender or food processor, combine the olive oil, lemon juice, basil, honey, pepper, salt, and garlic and blend until fully combined and bright green in color. Transfer to a bowl or jar, cover with plastic wrap, and refrigerate until ready to use. The dressing will keep in the refrigerator for up to 3 days.

Once the vegetables have cooled, cut the corn kernels from the cobs and cut the onion quarters into small pieces. Add to a large bowl with the remaining charred vegetables and the baby arugula, cherry tomatoes, and goat cheese. Drizzle with several spoonfuls of the dressing and toss well.

Serve the salad with the remaining dressing alongside.

Enjoy!

Farro Lentil Salad

Ingredients Needed

for 4 servings

3 ½ cups farro (350 g), cooked

1 ½ cups lentils (300 g), cooked

1 cup grape tomato (150 g), halved

1 cup cucumber (135 g), diced

½ cup yellow bell pepper (50 g), diced

½ cup red bell pepper (50 g)

⅓ cup fresh parsley (15 g), chopped

⅓ cup olive oil (80 mL)

2 tablespoons red wine vinegar

2 tablespoons lemon juice

1 teaspoon dijon mustard

1 clove garlic, minced

1 teaspoon italian seasoning

½ teaspoon salt

¼ teaspoon pepper

fresh arugula, to taste, optional

How To Prepare :

In a medium bowl, combine the farro, lentils, tomatoes, cucumber, yellow pepper, red pepper, and parsley.

In a liquid measuring cup or small bowl, combine the olive oil, red wine vinegar, lemon juice, Dijon mustard, garlic, Italian seasoning, salt, and pepper, and whisk until well-combined.

Pour the vinaigrette over the farro salad and toss until well-combined.

Distribute the farro salad into airtight containers with the arugula, if using. Refrigerate for up to 5 days.

Enjoy!

Grilled Corn Summer Pasta Salad

Ingredients

for 6 servings

Pasta Salad

2 ears corn

olive oil, for brushing

8 oz dried orecchiette pasta (225 g), cooked according to package instructions

2 cups cherry tomato (400 g)

½ cup red onion (75 g), diced

1 avocado, diced

Cilantro-Lime Vinaigrette

1 ½ cups fresh cilantro (60 g)

⅓ cup olive oil (80 mL)

3 tablespoons lime juice

1 clove garlic, roughly chopped

½ teaspoon chili powder

2 teaspoons honey

salt, to taste

pepper, to taste

How To Prepare :

Microwave the corn on a microwave-safe plate on high for 7 minutes. Remove from the microwave, and grip the corn with a dish towel. Then cut off the bottom end with a serrated knife. Slide the corn out of the husk. It should come out fairly easily with none of the silky string mess.

Brush the corn with olive oil, then place on a cast iron grill pan or outdoor grill over medium-high heat. Grill for 5-6 minutes on each side, until the kernels are slightly charred.

Insert the narrow end of an ear of corn into the center hole of a bundt pan. Holding the corn steady with one hand, saw off the kernels with a serrated knife. The kernels will fall into the pan for easy collection.

Make the cilantro-lime vinaigrette: Combine the cilantro, olive oil, lime juice, garlic, chili powder, honey, salt, and pepper in a food processor and blend until smooth.

In a large bowl, add the pasta, corn, tomatoes, red onion, avocado, and vinaigrette, and mix until well-combined.

Enjoy!

Strawberry Poppy Seed Salad With Grilled Chicken

Ingredients

for 1 serving

Poppy Seed Dressing

2 tablespoons olive oil

3 tablespoons nonfat greek yogurt

2 tablespoons red wine vinegar

1 tablespoon lemon juice

1 teaspoon honey

1 teaspoon poppy seed

½ teaspoon dijon mustard

¼ teaspoon salt

¼ teaspoon ground black pepper

1 boneless, skinless chicken breast, sliced into 1/2-inch (1-cm) pieces

½ teaspoon salt

¼ teaspoon ground black pepper

¼ teaspoon paprika

2 teaspoons olive oil

2 cups baby spinach (80 g)

½ cup strawberry (75 g), hulled and sliced

½ avocado, sliced

1 tablespoon sliced almond, toasted

How To Prepare :

In a bowl, add the olive oil, Greek yogurt, red wine vinegar, lemon juice, honey, poppy seeds, mustard, salt, and pepper in a small bowl and whisk until emulsified.

Season the chicken with salt, pepper, and paprika.

Heat olive oil in a pan over medium heat. Once the oil begins to shimmer, add the chicken and cook until browned on both sides, about 4 minutes per side.

Once cooled, slice the chicken on a cutting board.

Toss spinach, strawberries, avocado, almonds, and sliced chicken together in a large bowl and drizzle with poppy seed dressing.

Enjoy!

Avocado & Yogurt Chicken Salad

Ingredients

for 2 servings

Chicken Salad

1 cup cooked chicken (125 g), chopped or shredded

¼ cup celery (55 g), chopped

¼ cup red onion (35 g), diced

2 tablespoons fresh parsley, chopped

1 lime, juiced

salt, to taste

pepper, to taste

Mayonnaise Substitute Options (choose one)*

1 ripe avocado, mashed

¾ cup nonfat greek yogurt (215 g)

How To Prepare :

Add mashed avocado (or non-fat Greek yogurt), cooked chicken, celery, red onion, parsley, lime juice, salt, and pepper.

Stir until well combined.

Enjoy!

Hearty Roasted Veggie Salad

Ingredients Needed

for 4 servings

3 beets

1 cup olive oil (240 mL), divided

1 ½ teaspoons salt, divided

1 red onion, cut into wedges

4 carrots, peeled and chopped

2 parsnips, peeled, chopped

1 sweet potato, peeled, chopped

¾ teaspoon pepper, divided

2 tablespoons balsamic vinegar

1 tablespoon lemon juice

1 tablespoon dijon mustard

½ teaspoon garlic powder

3 tablespoons fresh parsley, chopped

6 cups mixed greens (600 g)

1 cup walnuts (100 g), chopped

½ cup crumbled feta cheese (55 g)

How To Prepare :

Preheat oven to 425°F (220°C).

On a cutting board, cut the root end of the beet so it lays flat on the surface. Place the beet on a piece of aluminum foil. Drizzle with 1 tablespoon of olive oil and season with ¼ teaspoon salt. Wrap the foil around the beet and pinch the top of the foil together until the beet is sealed in. Repeat with the other 2 beets.

On a sheet pan, place the onions, carrots, parsnips, and sweet potato.

Drizzle with 3 tablespoons olive oil and season with ½ teaspoon pepper and ½ teaspoon salt. Toss the the vegetables until coated and spread them evenly in the pan.

Create 3 circular spaces for the beets. Place the 3 beets on the pan.

Bake for 1 hour until with vegetables begin to crisp and caramelize.

In a large bowl, add ½ cup (120 ml) of olive oil, balsamic vinegar, lemon juice, Dijon mustard, and garlic powder, and whisk until emulsified. Add the parsley and season with salt and pepper, stirring to combine.

Add the mixed greens, roasted vegetables, and the beets to the bowl with the vinaigrette and toss until evenly incorporated.

Serve with walnuts and feta.

Enjoy!

Roasted Sweet Potato And Apple Salad

Ingredients Needed

for 2 servings

Cinnamon Apple Cider Vinaigrette

3 tablespoons olive oil

2 tablespoons apple cider vinegar

1 teaspoon honey

½ teaspoon dijon mustard

¼ teaspoon salt

¼ teaspoon ground black pepper

¼ teaspoon ground cinnamon

½ cup sweet potato (100 g), diced

1 boneless, skinless chicken breast

2 teaspoons olive oil

1 teaspoon salt

½ teaspoon ground black pepper

¼ teaspoon paprika

1 apple, cored and sliced

2 cups baby spinach (80 g)

2 tablespoons feta cheese, crumbled

2 tablespoons walnuts, toasted, unsalted, and chopped

How To Prepare :

Preheat oven to 400°F (200°C).

In a measuring cup, add the olive oil, apple cider vinegar, honey, mustard, salt, pepper, and cinnamon and whisk to combine.

Place sweet potatoes and chicken breast on a parchment paper-lined sheet tray and season with olive oil, salt, pepper, and paprika.

Bake until chicken is cooked through and sweet potatoes are tender, 15-18 minutes.

Slice the chicken breast.

Toss the sweet potatoes and sliced chicken with the sliced apples, feta, and walnuts and drizzle with vinaigrette.

Enjoy!

Southwestern Salad

Ingredients

for 1 serving

Dressing

½ avocado

1 lime, juiced

2 cloves garlic

½ teaspoon salt

½ cup water (120 mL)

Salad

½ green bell pepper, chopped

½ cup corn (85 g)

½ cup cherry tomato (100 g), halved

¼ cup quinoa (40 g), cooked

½ cup black beans (85 g)

1 cup spinach (40 g)

How To Prepare :

In a food processor, combine the avocado, lime juice, garlic, salt, and water. Pulse until smooth, then transfer to a large mason jar.

Add the bell pepper, corn, cherry tomatoes, quinoa, black beans, and spinach and screw on the lid.

Store in the refrigerator until ready to eat, up to 5 days.

Give the mason jar a good shake to mix and use a fork or spoon to stir as needed.

Enjoy!

Buttermilk-fried Chicken Salad

Ingredients Needed

for 4 servings

8 boneless, skinless chicken thighs

oil, for frying

10 oz spring mix green (285 g)

2 roma tomatoes, sliced

1 large cucumber, sliced

1 red onion, sliced thin

Buttermilk Marinade

2 cups buttermilk (480 mL)

1 teaspoon salt

1 teaspoon black pepper

½ teaspoon cayenne pepper

Dill Dressing

1 ½ cups plain greek yogurt (425 g)

3 tablespoons fresh dill, chopped

1 tablespoon garlic powder

2 tablespoons lemon juice

Seasoned Flour

2 cups all-purpose flour (250 g)

1 tablespoon salt

1 ½ teaspoons black pepper

1 teaspoon cayenne pepper

1 tablespoon garlic powder

How To Prepare :

In a medium bowl, combine all the buttermilk marinade ingredients. Toss in chicken thighs and marinate for at least one hour in the refrigerator.

In a small bowl, combine all the **Ingredients** for dill dressing. Cover and let sit for at least an hour in the refrigerator.

In a medium bowl, combine all **Ingredients** for seasoned flour.

Dip chicken in flour until chicken is completely covered. Repeat for all chicken thighs.

Heat the oil to 350°F (180°C) in a deep pot. Do not fill more than ½ full with oil.

Carefully fry chicken for roughly 7 minutes, or until cooked through (internal temperature reaches 165°F (75°C)) golden brown and crispy. Drain on a paper towel.

Layer a couple handfuls of spring mix greens on a plate. Add sliced tomatoes, cucumbers, and red onions. Top with fried chicken. Spoon the dill dressing on top of the salad.

Enjoy!

Summer Vegetable Pesto Ribbon Salad

Ingredients

for 4 servings

Salad

2 zucchinis

2 yellow squashes

2 carrots

2 cups grape tomato (400 g)

olive oil, for drizzling

salt, to taste

pepper, to taste

Pesto

2 cups fresh basil (80 g)

1 cup fresh parsley (35 g)

½ cup cashews (65 g)

1 clove garlic

½ teaspoon salt

¼ teaspoon pepper

1 tablespoon lemon juice

½ cup olive oil (120 mL)

How To Prepare :

Cut the ends off the zucchini. With a vegetable peeler, shave off as many thin slices as possible and transfer a large bowl. Repeat with the yellow squash and carrots.

Place the grape tomatoes between 2 large plates or tupperware lids. Press down, securing the tomatoes in place, and use a long, sharp knife to slice the tomatoes in half. Add to the bowl with the shaved vegetables.

Drizzle olive oil over the vegetables and season with salt and pepper. Toss to combine.

Make the pesto: Add the basil, parsley, cashews, garlic, salt, pepper, lemon juice, and olive oil to a food processor and process until smooth.

Spoon the pesto onto the shaved vegetables and mix well with tongs until fully coated and serve. Enjoy!

Ratatouille Salad

Ingredients

for 2 servings

olive oil, for cooking

1 large eggplant, or 2 small, cubed

salt, to taste

pepper, to taste

1 red bell pepper, seeded and chopped

yellow bell pepper, seeded and chopped

1 small white onion, chopped

2 cloves garlic, minced

1 yellow squash, sliced

1 zucchini, sliced

1 tablespoon fresh thyme, chopped

3 roma tomatoes, diced

½ lemon, juiced

1 cup white quinoa (170 g), uncooked

2 ½ cups water (600 mL)

1 tablespoon fresh basil, chopped

How To Prepare :

Heat a bit of olive oil in a large skillet over medium heat. Add the eggplant, season with salt and pepper, and cook, stirring occasionally, until golden brown and softened, 5-10 minutes. Remove from the pan and drain on paper towels.

Heat more oil in the pan, then add the bell peppers. Cook, stirring occasionally, until softened, 2-3 minutes.

Add the onion and garlic and cook, stirring, until the onions are soft and golden, about 3 minutes. Remove the peppers and onions from the pan.

Add the yellow squash and zucchini, season with salt and pepper, and cook squash have cooked down a bit, about 5 minutes.

Add the thyme and tomatoes, season with more salt, then add the lemon juice. Increase the heat to high and cook until mixture is sizzling. Cook, stirring occasionally, until the tomatoes start to release their juices, about 2 minutes.

Return the eggplant and pepper mixture to the pan, stir to combine, then remove the pan from the heat.

Add the quinoa and water to a large skillet and stir to combine. Bring to a boil, then cover and reduce the heat to low. Simmer until the liquid is absorbed, about 20 minutes.

Spoon the vegetables over quinoa and sprinkle the basil on top. Serve warm.

Enjoy!

Kale & Sweet Potato Salad

Ingredients Needed

for 4 servings

1 ½ cups sweet potato (300 g), diced

½ teaspoon garlic powder

2 teaspoons paprika

salt, to taste

pepper, to taste

olive oil, to taste

½ cup pumpkin seeds (65 g)

2 teaspoons chili powder

2 tablespoons maple syrup, divided

½ cup tahini (110 g)

1 ½ tablespoons lemon juice

3 tablespoons water

1 bunch kale, stemmed and torn into large pieces

3 cups quinoa (510 g)

½ cup red onion (75 g), diced

How To Prepare :

Preheat the oven to 375°F (190°C).

Add the sweet potatoes to a baking sheet. Sprinkle with the garlic powder, paprika, salt, and pepper, and drizzle with olive oil. Toss until the sweet potato is well-coated in the spices, then spread out evenly. Bake for 15 minutes, or until tender.

In a small bowl, add the pumpkin seeds, chili powder, 1 tablespoon maple syrup, and salt, and mix until well-combined. Spread the pumpkin seeds out on a baking sheet so they're not touching each other.

Add to the oven with the sweet potato and bake for 10 minutes, stirring halfway through, until toasted.

In a liquid measuring cup, combine the tahini, remaining tablespoon of maple syrup, lemon juice, salt, and pepper. Mix well, then add 1 tablespoon of water at a time until desired consistency is reached.

In a large bowl, drizzle the kale with olive oil. Massage with your hands until the kale is tender and has reduced in volume by about a third.

Add the quinoa, roasted sweet potatoes, red onion, and pumpkin seeds. Drizzle with tahini dressing and toss well.

Serve with more dressing if desired.

Enjoy!

Protein-Packed Roasted Vegetable Salad

Ingredients

for 1 serving

Dressing

2 tablespoons hummus

1 tablespoon lemon juice

1 tablespoon olive oil

1 teaspoon dried thyme

½ teaspoon salt

½ teaspoon pepper

½ teaspoon water

Salad

nonstick cooking spray

½ cup broccoli floret (75 g)

½ cup chickpeas (100 g)

½ cup brussel sprout (50 g), halved

½ cup sweet potato (100 g), peeled and chopped

½ cup tofu (125 g), pressed and chopped

¼ cup olive oil (60 mL)

½ teaspoon salt

½ teaspoon pepper

1 tablespoon chili powder

1 cup spinach (40 g)

How To Prepare :

Preheat the oven to 400°F (200°C). Grease a baking sheet with nonstick spray.

Reserve a few broccoli florets, then place the remaining broccoli, chickpeas, Brussels sprouts, sweet potato, and tofu on the baking sheet in individual piles. Drizzle with the olive oil and season with salt, pepper, and chili powder. Bake for 25 minutes, until the vegetables are tender and the tofu is browned.

Make the dressing: In a large mason jar, combine the hummus, lemon juice, olive oil, thyme, salt, pepper, and water. Stir to combine.

Add the reserved raw broccoli, the roasted broccoli, sweet potato, chickpeas, Brussels sprouts, tofu, and spinach and screw on the lid.

Store in the refrigerator until ready to eat, up to 5 days.

Give the mason jar a good shake to mix and use a fork or spoon to stir as needed.

Enjoy!

Honey Mustard Chicken Salad

Ingredients Needed

for 4 servings

⅓ cup honey (115 g)

¼ cup dijon mustard (65 g)

2 tablespoons olive oil

2 cloves garlic, minced

2 teaspoons salt

1 teaspoon pepper

4 boneless, skinless chicken thighs

¼ cup bacon (60 g), chopped

4 cups romaine lettuce (300 g), chopped

1 cup cherry tomatoes (200 g), halved

¼ red onion, sliced

1 avocado, pitted and sliced

How To Prepare :

In a small bowl or liquid measuring cup, mix the honey, mustard, oil, garlic, salt, and pepper.

Place the chicken thighs in a dish and pour the marinade over the chicken, reserving half for later.

Flip the chicken thighs over, fully covering them in the marinade.

Cover the dish with plastic wrap and refrigerate for 30 minutes to an hour.

Heat a large skillet over medium heat, and place the chicken thighs in the pan.

Cook for five minutes on each side, or until the chicken is cooked through.

Remove the chicken and set aside.

Wipe the pan clean and place back on the heat.

Add the chopped bacon to the pan and cook until crispy, about ten minutes.

Transfer the bacon to a paper towel-lined plate to drain.

Add three tablespoons of water to the reserved marinade and stir to combine.

Slice the chicken into strips.

Add the romaine, cherry tomatoes, red onion, avocado, cooked bacon, and chicken to a bowl and drizzle with the remaining honey mustard dressing.

Enjoy!

Avocado Quinoa Power Salad

Ingredients Needed

for 6 servings

Salad

2 cups water (480 mL)

salt, to taste

1 cup quinoa (170 g), rinsed

2 cups fresh spinach (80 g), roughly chopped

1 large cucumber, diced

4 roma tomatoes, diced

2 ripe avocados, pits removed and diced

1 lemon, juiced

4 tablespoons extra virgin olive oil

pepper, to taste

How To Prepare :

In a small saucepan, bring the water and a pinch of salt to a boil. Add the quinoa, cover, and simmer for 15 minutes, or until the water is absorbed. Transfer to a medium bowl to cool to room temperature, then fluff the quinoa.

Refrigerate the quinoa for 20 minutes.

Add the spinach, cucumber, tomatoes, and avocado to the bowl of quinoa and mix to combine.

Add the lemon juice, olive oil, salt, and pepper, and mix well.

Enjoy!

CHAPTER 8
In Summary

In the labyrinth of medical conditions, Addison's Disease stands as a rare yet formidable adversary, quietly affecting the lives of those it touches. Our exploration of this condition has unveiled its enigmatic nature, from the subtle onset of symptoms to the potential life-threatening crises it can precipitate. In traversing the landscape of Addison's Disease, we have journeyed through its etiology, manifestations, diagnostic challenges, and treatment modalities, each step revealing the complexity of its management and the resilience required to confront it.

Central to navigating Addison's Disease is the importance of early recognition and diagnosis. The elusive nature of its symptoms, often mimicking other more common ailments, underscores the necessity for heightened clinical suspicion. Timely identification not only facilitates prompt intervention to prevent adrenal crises but also lays the foundation for tailored treatment strategies aimed at mitigating symptoms and optimizing quality of life.

Yet, the journey of those living with Addison's Disease extends far beyond the confines of medical intervention. It is a journey marked by resilience, adaptation, and unwavering perseverance. Coping with the uncertainties of a chronic illness, managing daily medication regimens, and navigating the emotional rollercoaster that accompanies a life-altering diagnosis demand a holistic approach to care. The significance of psychological support, patient education, and community resources cannot be overstated in fostering resilience and empowering individuals to thrive despite the challenges they face.

While medical science has made significant strides in unraveling the mysteries of Addison's Disease, formidable challenges persist. Disparities in access to healthcare, gaps in provider knowledge, and the need for continued research to elucidate underlying mechanisms and develop novel therapies remain formidable hurdles. As we stand on the precipice of progress, it is imperative that we unite in our commitment to advancing the understanding and management of Addison's

Disease, ensuring that no individual faces this condition alone or without hope for a brighter tomorrow.

In the tapestry of human experience, Addison's Disease occupies a unique thread, weaving its way through the lives of those it touches. Through our collective efforts—patients, caregivers, healthcare professionals, and researchers alike—we can illuminate this thread, transforming it from a source of darkness into a beacon of resilience and hope. In the pages of this book, we have embarked on a journey through the complexities of Addison's Disease, shedding light on its impact and offering insights into its management. May this knowledge serve as a compass, guiding us toward a future where the burden of Addison's

Disease is alleviated, and the resilience of those affected shines brightly for all to see.

Printed in Great Britain
by Amazon